"I had the privilege of serving as chaplain to Aud[...] many months/years they were in and out of Chil[...] Hospital & Medical Center in Omaha, NE. Brigitte's book is an amazing, thoughtful account of their experience and the many things they learned in caring for their daughter. Their strength and faith are evident throughout. It is an excellent source of information and helpful advice for any parent who has a child with a chronic medical condition."

Chaplain Sheila Mee, DMin, BCC, CHTP
Supervisor - Pastoral & Spiritual Care,
Children's Hospital and Medical Center of Omaha

"Transplantation is a journey – and everyone's journey is unique. Often, it is not an easy road to travel with many twists and turns and ups and downs. The journey is certainly made easier with supportive friends, family members and close communications/collaborations with members of the medical staffs. In this book I find a message of hope, courage, determination and the message that staying positive and focused helps out even in the most challenging times. No matter what issues a parent or family member of a child undergoing transplantation might face, this book provides many creative ideas on ways to navigate through the process of transplantation. As said in a Chinese Proverb, 'A journey of a thousand miles must begin with the first step.' May this book provide you with many 'first steps' on your own journey."

Laurel Williams, RN, MSN, CCTC
Liver and Intestinal Transplant Coordinator,
University of Nebraska Medical Center

"When a loved one, particularly a child, is facing a chronic critical illness, it's easy to go into melt-down mode. Through experience, Brigitte has learned the ins and outs of long hospitalizations, how to turn a home into a hospital-like setting (and vice versa) and how to forge through the mind-numbing ups and downs of having a very seriously ill child. This is a great read for those experiencing a serious medical situation or for those on the sidelines who want to help but don't know how."

Michele Rutledge, a lifelong friend who lost her father to cancer after a lengthy battle

Just So
You Know ...
For Parents

Just So
You Know ...
For Parents

Brigitte D. Crist

Published by Pretty Prairie Press

ISBN-10: 0615753051
ISBN-13: 978-0615753058

Cover Design by Karis Gensch
Cover Photo and Other Photos by Brigitte Crist
Cover Models: Sherri Kahrs and Terri Dugger

Resource for terms/definitions: Julie Becklun and Laurel Williams

To schedule Brigitte as a speaker, or for any questions/comments,
she may be contacted at:

prettyprairie.net / parent2parent

To register as an organ and tissue donor, visit
donatelife.net today!

Dedicated to *Audrey Beth* ...

Our daughter, and the reason for this book: For allowing me such a brave example to share with other children, who are living with medical challenges, and with their families...who could use a touch of your courage and joy right now.

Also ...

To all of the families who have committed their love, time, energy, and resources to doing everything possible to help their children who are fighting for their lives.

Table of Contents

Acknowledgements

𝒯here are a number of people whom I would like to recognize; they have each played a vital role in Audrey's care and recovery, and the well-being of our entire family. Included are our team of supporters, the staff who cared for Audrey, and so many unsung heroes...

Our Team of Supporters:

- Our Family – for your support and presence throughout our crisis
- Our Friends
- Our Churches
- The readers of our "Audrey Updates" and Carepage – an extensive group of family members, friends, friends of friends, multiple churches and Bible study groups that reach around the globe.
- Our Hospital Community – other patients, along with *your* families and friends.

We thank you for your encouragement and prayer support, we appreciate your help with meals, babysitting, yard work, visits and gifts, packages via the mail, and countless notes and phone calls checking in on us and cheering us on!

Staff Members at Children's Hospital and Medical Center of Omaha and The Nebraska Medical Center:

- Doctors and Surgeons:
  - Dr. Stephen Raynor and his team and office staff in Pediatric Surgery at Children's Hospital
  - The Gastroenterology Team at Children's Hospital
  - Dr. Kalid Awad, and the Team of Neonatologists at Children's Hospital
  - Liver Transplant Team at the Nebraska Medical Center
  - Dr. Thomas Byrne and Dr. Rebecca Reddy, our Pediatricians

- Nursing Staff and Care Partners/Techs
- Participating specialists, i.e. Oncologists, Neurologists, Infectious Disease, Radiology Staff and Lab Technicians; Occupational and Physical Therapists, Respiratory Therapists, Pharmacy, Child Life and Child Development personnel, namely Jen Tyler and Kathy Walburn; Social Workers, and Pastoral Care; and all of the personnel who were always kind and welcoming to us with friendly smiles, a helping hand or a word of encouragement or advice: This includes but is not exclusive to those in the Resource Room, Admission, doctors' offices, ladies at the front desk and other receptionists, the gift shop, the coffee shop, the cafeteria, and every department or staff member we rubbed shoulders with in the hallway or elevator.
- Other Support Staff, i.e. Housekeeping and Food Services
- Children's Home Health Care in Omaha: For late night replacements of malfunctioning pumps, special orders, friendly and first-rate service!
- Rainbow House of Omaha
- The Make-A-Wish Foundation of Omaha
- Give Kids The World Village in Kissimmee, Florida
- The Donate Life Organization
- Carepages

And Last, but Certainly not Least ...

For those friends and family members who encouraged me in my endeavor to write this book and who helped in the editing, as well as contributing your endorsements, ideas, and much valued critique:

- My Husband, Dallas
- My Mom and Dad, Sonja and Bill Randall
- Healthcare professionals, whom I also call friends: Dr. Stephen Raynor, Julie Becklun, Lesa Grovas, and Laurel Williams
- Other dear friends, Beth Crichton and Michele Rutledge
- Dr. Rhonda Wright – Pediatric Neurology, Children's Hospital and Medical Center of Omaha
- Arlen Busenitz - Publishing Consultant, Grow4Success.com

A Note to You, the Reader…

From my spacious hospital room window, while recovering from Audrey's birth, I enjoyed a marvelous view of trees in full bloom throughout the neighborhood below. *It was springtime …* As the days, weeks, and months passed, work began on the hospital grounds – planting flowers for the coming summer. My mom and I watched this progression from spring to summer, and into the fall, as mums replaced the fading summer growth. Then winter set in and blanketed the mums.

Meanwhile, in NICU *(Neonatal Intensive Care Unit)*, as *Audrey* was recovering, she graduated from an open-style incubator, to an enclosed incubator, to a first-stage crib, to a full-sized crib. As she continued to heal, grow and develop in those beds, she grew out of her newborn outfits *(which she rarely was able to wear anyway)* into her six-month clothes, then into her nine-month snowsuit, which became her new *"going home"* dress! These were just some ways we measured the passage of time. It took us a couple of months to learn not to ask the question, *"When…?"*.

This book has been several years in the making. It started with journaling during Audrey's hospital stays. I finally began work on the manuscript a couple of years ago. It has taken the full two years or so to take it from manuscript form to a published work. Within that time, I have edited, revised, added and omitted; our family has made four moves, some of them cross-country (not including the moves *"pre-manuscript!"*); I have homeschooled and worked part-time somewhere in there! Though I have set and reset deadlines for my book countless times, I'm glad to have started and completed this work. Besides a great sense of accomplishment, I hope my words will truly prove helpful in some way to you; because that is ultimately the reason for this book!

Sincerely,

Brigitte Crist

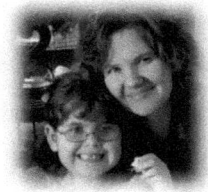

Forward

$\mathcal{I}$ remember the day I met Brigitte and Audrey Crist as if it were yesterday, but in many ways it feels like a lifetime ago. It was not long after I had started working with the pediatric surgeons at Childrens' Hospital of Omaha. The secretary advised me that Audrey was in the lobby with an enterocutaneous fistula. Since both of the surgeons were in the operating room, it was my responsibility to go and see what I could do to help. I had never addressed such a diagnosis before. So as I rode down in the elevator, I reviewed how one might manage an "enterocutaneous fistula," and how I would find them. I imagined I would recognize Brigitte as the panicked mother! This was not the case at all. In the lobby, I was greeted by a radiant, smiling woman, confidently holding an adorable toddler. Brigitte's first words to me were *"Just so you know ..."*

After that, the *"Just so you know"* statements continued, but they were not from Brigitte - they were from Audrey, as she taught our surgical team how to do dressing changes, or as she explained the needs of a preschooler to a team of surgical residents. Those days were filled with some of the most valuable lessons - lessons learned from stopping and listening to a spontaneous child and her remarkable mother. Those days were also filled with miraculous operations, time consuming dressing changes, bad news, long waits, and changes in care providers and hospitals, as the family went for transplant. But, as a family, they got stronger and made it through.

Throughout it all, Brigitte had a presence of peace about her that few other parents exhibit. She worked endlessly to ensure that Audrey had a life in the hospital, not just an existence. She kept a journal, and continuously seemed to have a list of sincere questions to clarify her understanding of the medical decisions being made in regards to Audrey.

On a recent visit to our hospital, Brigitte shared with me that she was planning to write this book, in hopes that her experiences with Audrey would be of help to another parent. I was very excited to know others would have the chance to learn from Brigitte. I felt she had so much to offer other parents in similar situations. As you progress in your own journey with an ill child, may the guidance provided here by Brigitte encourage you and give you peace.

Lesa Grovas, MN, APRN-NP
Pediatric Nurse Practitioner

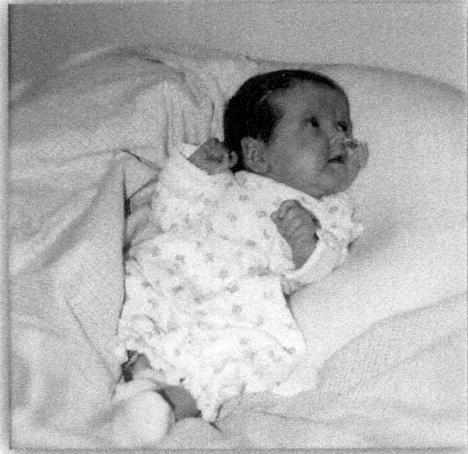

Introduction ...

My husband, Dallas, and I were adjusting to life as newlyweds. Then came the exciting news that we were expecting our first child. Four months into the pregnancy, a routine sonogram showed a defect in our baby's development. Two and a half short months later, our daughter Audrey was born - seven weeks prematurely. For the next nine months we lived in the Neonatal Intensive Care Unit (known as NICU), as our baby battled to overcome continual medical challenges.

Audrey's diagnosis, known as "gastroschisis," is a birth defect that occurs early in pregnancy. Her body cavity failed to developed around her bowel, leaving the organs outside and exposed to the amniotic fluid. She was taken into surgery shortly after birth to place her bowel back into the body cavity. For the next several years, related complications caused further surgeries and extended hospital stays.

Ultimately, Audrey received a multi-organ transplant at age four *(small bowel, liver, and pancreas)*. I am very pleased to announce that, as I write this, she is now a happy and thriving nine year old!

Until about age five, however, Audrey had spent as much time in the hospital as she had at home. We came to refer to the hospital as our "vacation home." When the nurses received word that we were back, they would make the extra effort to get us a "penthouse suite" if available ... or at least a room with a view!

It has been a grueling journey - we have dealt with despairing news, fear and uncertainty, disappointments and frustrations, an overload of stress, and sheer anxiety over the possibility of losing our daughter. Audrey has dealt with all of the above along with extreme pain and discomfort. Just the lack of control we had over her circumstances *and* ours was difficult to manage much of the time.

Throughout the months we logged as "inpatient " (sometimes "*im*patient!"), we learned how to cope with Audrey's condition and her prognosis, as well as making our home in a hospital room. It became our way of life ... living for months on end in the hospital, packing and unpacking - from home to hospital and hospital to home. We had no choice but to adapt and to continue living our lives. Some days that meant a trip to the gift shop to buy Dr. Raynor some taffy, or adventures to the "river" to throw pennies. Other days we just held on and survived. One year, we had spent so much time in the hospital that the first opportunity we were able to escape out of town for a long weekend of fun, Audrey kept referring to the hotel as the "hospital!" As I share with you a portion of our story along with a collection of survival tips, I hope that you may find courage to keep going in your present circumstances.

Perhaps you will find some of these pages to be enjoyable reading during a coffee break, while you digest other pages during the many, *many* opportunities you will have to develop the virtue of patience!

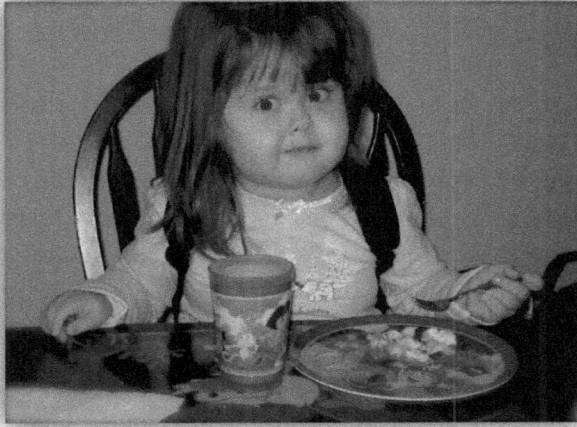

Chapter 1

Why I Write to You

"If I can help you get through one more day with a little more hope, this book will have been worth it to me!"

*A*s I begin, I'd like to share with you the inspiration behind the title of this book. A few years ago, Audrey went through a stage of using the phrase, *"Just so ya know..."* Being the helpful and engaging little girl that she is, she was ever anxious to keep people, namely medical staff, "in the know." *"Just so ya know, I am allergic to . . .", "Just so ya know, I like my temperature taken under my arm . . .", "Just so ya know, we use adhesive remover (the kind that smells like oranges)."* And so the phrase was coined.

Like my daughter, I want to help and pass along to you some ideas that led our family through difficult times, and lent value to our experience. We realized how important it was to make the best of our circumstances, for us as parents *and* for our daughter as the patient.

To see that she received the best care possible, we had to be on top of our game. This meant taking care of ourselves and of our marriage, while incorporating as much "normalcy" into Audrey's life and her routine as was allowed. We also quickly learned that *we* were part of the team of people who would see Audrey through her struggles and ensure her successful recovery and return home, if possible, to life as it should be for her and for us.

The First Few Years, Condensed -

To set the stage for the chapters that follow, I will share a bit of Audrey's history with you. And as I mentioned in *The Introduction*, our story starts at the very beginning of the formation of our family. The complications surrounding my pregnancy caused our baby to go into distress, resulting in her early delivery, on April 15, 2003. We spent a little over nine months in the NICU at Children's Hospital and Medical Center of Omaha. Audrey's initial surgery led to numerous other operations.

Due to their fragile condition, the loops of intestine were damaged easily during surgery. In addition, scar tissue that formed with each invasion into the abdominal cavity continued to thicken and tighten around the bowel, adding stress to the organ. This led to strictures *(narrowings)*, and contributed to the perforations *(holes)*, which would become fistulas, openings in the bowel breaking through at the surface of the skin. It was a vicious cycle for several months - a fistula or stricture forming, which would call for emergency surgery; then a return trip to the operating room would be required again because of further strictures or fistulas.

Audrey spent her first summer months with an open wound across the width of her belly, containing two fistulas that emptied contents from her bowel *(intestines)* on the exposed skin around her wound. It was a challenge to figure out the best way to absorb this drainage, so that bile and other gastric juices draining from the holes in her bowel wouldn't burn and eat away at her skin. The situation required her to be on intravenous nutrition *(known as TPN)* for most of this time. Her doctors, also posing as ingenious inventors and engineers, created ways of supplementing her nutrition with the milk that I pumped and with formula by administering it through a feeding tube inserted into one of the fistulas. They were constantly solving one problem directly after another.

Around Christmas time, we started seeing a potential end to our hospital stay - the fistulas were healing, and no new ones had formed. By the third week of January, we were finally able to take Audrey home for the first time; she was over nine months old. She continued on TPN as we began teaching her how to eat. By her first birthday, she was no longer on TPN, and was eating regular table food, though most of it was lost with perpetual reflux, as she spit it back up!

A Move (or two) Cross-Country ...

In May, we moved from Omaha, and took up temporary residence with my parents in Wichita, KS, while Dallas was transferred to a job on the east coast. Audrey and I spent the summer in Wichita, wrapped up some doctors' appointments in Omaha, and then joined Dallas in Virginia in the fall. We were there until the middle of November, when Dallas got word on a Thursday that he was to be in Miami by Monday to start on another project

We lasted in Miami for about five months - until March of 2005, when Audrey developed another fistula. She was in the children's hospital in Miami for a few days until we could make arrangements to transport her back to Omaha.

In Omaha, she was admitted to Children's Hospital, this time in the Pediatric Unit instead of the NICU; it felt strangely like coming back home! She underwent surgery to repair the fistula, and turned two years old during her stay.

About six weeks after our arrival, she was discharged, Dallas found work again in Omaha, and we moved into a home. Around the middle of the summer, she developed another red area on her belly. We kept an eye on it, and as it spread and became darker in color, we notified the doctors. They took her into the OR *(operating room)* to have a central line *(catheter)* inserted into a vein and put her back on TPN, making her NPO *(meaning no food by mouth)*. The first of September, the surgical team operated, repairing the fistula. She healed quickly, with no complications, and we were on our way home within a month.

Another Birthday without Cake ...
(Her Third so Far!)

We made it through the fall, winter, and part of the spring without any hospital stays. Then around her third birthday in April, another protrusion on her abdomen appeared. This time it wasn't red, but rather a little bump. The doctors had her admitted, and after examining the area and taking X-rays, they concluded that it probably was not a fistula, so they sent us home. A week or two later, the area started getting red.

We had her examined once again, and they realized that, indeed, it was the start of a fistula. So they inserted another central line, put her on TPN and made her NPO ... Sounds like déjà vu, doesn't it? Surgery was scheduled for May 31st, and they sent us home for about a month until then.

Audrey was taken into surgery on May 31st for a fistula repair as well as a procedure to take care of her reflux problem, which was causing her to spit up on a regular basis. The surgeries went well, and Audrey spent some time in the PICU (Pediatric Intensive Care Unit) before being transferred to the Pediatric floor for the remainder of her stay. She spent six months inpatient, as she endured further complications with fistulas, strictures, lazy bowel, line infections, etc. We spent the entire summer and well into the fall. There was no swimming or running barefoot in the grass, no swinging or catching fireflies, no days in the park. A construction company was making use of the hospital's only playground - to store their equipment. We had to make our own fun!

A Plan for Audrey's G.I. System –

During that six-month stint, we had met with the surgeon and the gastrointestinal doctor about options to treat Audrey's complicated GI (gastrointestinal) system. From birth, Audrey's GI tract wasn't healthy. The initial inflammation from exposure to the amniotic fluid had contributed significantly to the ongoing problems. The bowels were fragile, and tore easily. As I mentioned before, the subsequent and frequent surgeries created more and more adhesions (scar tissue). The resulting strictures challenged the passage of solids through the bowel.

The issues at hand were the following: How many more surgeries would her bowel handle? How much IV access did she have left for lines? With every bowel surgery, she required a central or PICC line for TPN for nutrition post-surgery until her bowels were ready to digest food. She had received so many lines already that most of her veins weren't in a condition to be accessed anymore.

The subject of small bowel transplant was presented in this meeting. When I had asked her surgeon about the option of a transplant just a few months previous, his reply had been a resounding *"absolutely not!"* A transplant would be *only* the last resort. It now looked like we had arrived at the "last resort." And a hospital stay would be the only resort accommodations we'd be enjoying for awhile!

The bowel contains the majority of the body's immune system. To replace it with a foreign organ, and then administer drugs to suppress *(or lower)* the immune system sounded like a death wish to me! The practice of such a procedure is one of the newest in the field of organ transplants. At the time of Audrey's transplant in 2008, the surgery was only about 10 years old - a *very risky* procedure ... but one that she desperately needed to save her life!

No conclusions resulted from this meeting, just options to consider; we would allow some time to pass to see what Audrey's bowels decided for us. So she was discharged from the hospital shortly before Thanksgiving, coming home once again on TPN and a feeding tube.

She tolerated very low enteral tube feeds *(formula was fed through a tube inserted into her stomach)* and even less table food, so she wasn't able to enjoy much of the Thanksgiving feast. She still had a constricted area that didn't allow for much food to pass through if it wasn't broken down quite a bit. Management of her central line was tricky, as it was inserted near the groin area. We had to be very careful about stool and wet diapers saturating the dressing and introducing infection to the insertion site.

In fact, just weeks after being home, Audrey contracted a line infection, which landed her back in the hospital. She was treated with antibiotics and then released to go home to complete her antibiotic regimen outpatient. We had to learn how to use another pump designed for home use. To say I was stressed at this point is an understatement! We had just spent six months living in the hospital; I was trying to adjust to life back at home with a new routine; and was now responsible for the management of her five or six oral medications, which were given several times a day; also her feeding tube, TPN, central line care, and now two IV antibiotics.

I was exceedingly paranoid about accessing her line to administer these medications. With each access, we ran the risk of introducing more germs to her line. When cleaning her ports *(the points of access on a central line)*, we had to follow protocol very closely. Central line infections are serious matters, which can even be fatal!

I wasn't used to the med pumps either. I got so flustered one day that I gave her the wrong antibiotic at the wrong time. I was so glad Dallas was home to calm me down and tell me it was going to be okay.

Just another Hospital Stay -
(Racking up our VIP credits!)

In January, Audrey spent three weeks in the hospital with a virus or the flu that had caused a high fever. Part of that time, I was also sick with the flu, and her nurses were caring for two patients, since I was too sick to get out of bed and drive home!

After this, she stayed out of the hospital for about six months. In July, the portion of upper bowel, which had been an area of concern the previous year, became more narrowed, preventing hardly any food, including liquids, from passing downstream. Audrey's abdomen had become very swollen and hard, causing her a great deal of pain and discomfort. The doctor stopped her tube feedings, returned her to full TPN, and scheduled her for surgery to take care of the stricture.

The "Big Surgery" ...

Audrey was scheduled for surgery on August 20th. We were now in the year 2007,and Audrey was four. This was to be the "big" surgery, as the location of the stricture was underneath layers of adhesions *(scar tissue)* that would have to be meticulously cut away from her bowels– I liken it to trying to carve fat off a steak without cutting into the steak! She was in the OR for 13 hours; and then the nightmare began. Her bowel began leaking from damaged areas that occurred in surgery. When removing scar tissue that is wrapped so tightly around loops of bowel, this kind of damage is inevitable. But with bowels that were weak and inflamed to start with, the outcome can be even worse.

Over the course of several days, perforations emerged, one right after the other, in her intestines. Audrey would have to be taken back into surgery several times for repair, or for placement of drainage tubes into these holes, in order to prevent the contents of her bowel from escaping into her body cavity around her belly and other organs. The repaired areas weren't holding together, and her intestines were falling apart.

The bowel is a very sensitive organ, and does not like being manipulated or messed with, much less so many times. By this point in her young life, Audrey had undergone about twenty-seven OR procedures on her abdomen and intestines.

The surgical team finally had no other option but to leave her belly open. They decided the best course of action would be to apply a wound vac dressing to the open wound, allowing the drainage to be suctioned out of her body cavity and her leaking bowel so that she wouldn't become septic, leading to blood poisoning. Bowel contents are very toxic to the body outside of the intestinal walls, and will lead to death if not contained. The steps toward bowel transplant then began.

A Transplant Underway ...

Audrey was sent home in November, and we waited for the call for her transplant, which came on January 3, 2008 - just under two months from our discharge from Children's. We made the trip down the street to the Nebraska Medical Center, and they prepared her for the procedure. The initial transplant was successful and she was recovering well. They had transplanted three organs: the liver, pancreas, and small bowel.

About two weeks post-transplant, Audrey became very sick. After consulting with numerous specialists from several departments, she was diagnosed with Graft vs. Host Disease, in which the newly *"grafted"* organs were attacking her body, the *host.* She was in a critical state for two to three weeks: She had aspirated, in which vomit entered into her lungs. Her lungs were unable to get rid of the fluid build-up, so she was put on a ventilator *(breathing machine)*. She then developed a fungus in her lungs, and the medical team was unsure whether she would be able to fight it off.

Over several days, a terrible red bumpy rash began covering her entire body, including her scalp. Her kidneys were shutting down, and they had to put her on dialysis treatments for about ten days to perform the function of her kidneys.

In addition, her new bowels had developed a tear, where a suture had torn apart, and they had to whisk her into emergency surgery to do a "wash out", flushing infection and bowel leakage from her body cavity. The surgical team was not sure whether she would pull out of it all - she was very sick, and it was a very dark time for us. We thought this really might be the end for our little girl ...

They raised the dosage of her steroid and anti-rejection medication to a significantly high level. She slowly began to show signs of improvement, and thankfully did recover!

A few weeks after her recovery from GVH *(Graft vs. Host)*, Audrey had a seizure that left her temporarily blind and unable to talk for almost ten days. With the seizure, Audrey had sustained damage to the nerve cell covering in her brain. This is defined as demyelination. At the time, it seemed surreal to me, like this couldn't really be happening. The neurosurgeon told us that she had never seen a brain scan like hers; it was just a cloudy gray. A normal CT scan should show the brain tissue as white in color. The neurosurgeon opted to do a brain biopsy on Audrey, hoping to discover the reason for the seizure activity and demyelination. The biopsy didn't offer any answers.

The transplant surgeons concluded the cause of the seizure to be a reaction to such a high dosage of her anti-rejection medication she was receiving during her case of Graft vs. Host Disease. They decided to switch her to a different anti-rejection medication. When her sight and speech finally returned, another brain scan indicated no demyelination at all - no sign of it! There were no explanations available, only sighs of relief ... and rejoicing! We knew some serious prayer had been answered!

Home Free!

On March 10th, we brought Audrey home. She was very weak. During her two month stay, besides the OR procedures, CT scans, and X-rays, Audrey had been sedated and on the ventilator for at least three of those weeks; so, she was bedridden a good part of her hospital stay. She was unable to walk on her own, and could barely hold up her head. It was difficult to lift a spoon to her mouth, and even harder to lift a cup. For the first couple of weeks, we had to either carry her or transport her in a wheel chair. This was a difficult task for us, as she had put on about 15 pounds of fluid – her small frame, formerly 45 pounds was now toting around more than 60 pounds!

After arriving home, Audrey immediately started outpatient physical and occupational therapy. Every session saw progress.

Less than a month after being discharged, she contracted Roto Virus in her bowel, which required another admission to the Med Center for about three weeks. So she spent her fifth year birthday in the hospital, once again unable to eat cake. I think this is why, rather than eating birthday cake, she came to prefer spending her birthdays with her nurses, her favorite people in the world!

In June, she took a tumble in her baby pool and hit her head, causing a seizure-like reaction. I called 911, and she was transported back to the Med Center via ambulance. The fall caused a bleed on her brain. She was more susceptible to a bleed like this, as she was on aspirin, along with a high dose of steroids. With a suppressed immune system *(due to the steroids)*, the white blood cells were slower to absorb any excess bleeding, and the aspirin aggravated the situation. We were so grateful and relieved that she recovered well, and was able to come home a few days later, with the intent of *staying* home for a long time – we'd had our fill of hospitals!

For the next year, Audrey continued in rehabilitation, we started homeschool, and took a trip to Disney World, sponsored by Make a Wish. She was on several medications, and still had an ostomy, which we managed at home; this required emptying and changing her ostomy bag. In April of the following year (2009), *after* her birthday, she had her ostomy removed, which meant that her colon was surgically reattached, and stool could now pass through her intestines the natural way! After some complications, she was released to go home - tube free, line free, bag free ... What a memorable event!

She has continued with good health and has made significant strides in regaining her strength. We've had a few minor bumps in the road, but overall, Audrey is thriving. A glimpse at this condensed version of Audrey's story will hopefully shed some light on our personal experience that led me to write this book.

As you continue through these pages, I will share how we tackled our own challenges and rallied our family together, and even came away with some cherished memories, great friends, and a much richer perspective on life in all of its ups and downs!

JSYK

On a Lighter Note...

We went through many frustrating moments just trying to carry on our lives within a clinical setting; however, we managed to approach some of the scenarios in our days with a bit of humor. The following is a sampling...

We knew it was time to go home when:

- The nurses no longer addressed us as "Mom" or "Dad", but rather on a first name basis.

- I started receiving an employee discount in the cafeteria.

- Our toddler knew her way around the hospital, and had friends in every corner!

- We found ourselves giving directions around the hospital to someone at least once a day!

- Our small daughter would give her IV pole a hug and kiss.

- Our child considered the playroom to be hers, and would scorn any other child who would play with *"her"* toys.

- I considered the waiting room to be *mine*, and would scorn anyone who would claim *"my"* post for the evening. And how dare they adjust the thermostat just after I had achieved that perfect temperature!

- The staff knew right where to find me if I wasn't at the bedside (i.e. one of my "offices" - a consultation room, waiting room...).

- I would no longer jump out of bed at early morning rounds - it was perfectly appropriate to carry on a conversation without even lifting my head from the pillow. And if I did rise, I was semi-comfortable being seen in my p.j.'s!

- I had claimed some ownership of the hospital property by weeding the flowerbeds while out for a stroll, tidying up the waiting room, straightening the items on the bookshelves, bringing in my own flower arrangement...

- We came to acknowledge staff members from other departments and floors with a certain familiarity after encountering each other so often in the elevators, hallways and cafeteria, and even between hospitals!

- One staff member, whom I had never met but had seen frequently in passing, had a dream about us one night!

- We reached the point where *we* were training the nurses on our child's care!

- The "Prox" card (for entry into our child's unit) wore an imprint in our back pockets.

- We reached a level of fluency in the medical jargon that used to cause us blank stares as parents new to the clinical world...*(and so had our toddler!)*

- I had earned my own frequent purchase card at the hospital coffee shop.

- We found ourselves sneaking down back hallways to avoid running into too many people we knew when we were in a hurry! *(I even considered donning shades in order to go unrecognized!)*

- Our child became bored with the same back hallways, because we had worn paths in the carpet from our countless adventures. We were out of new territory to explore; the same old routes had lost their wonder . . .

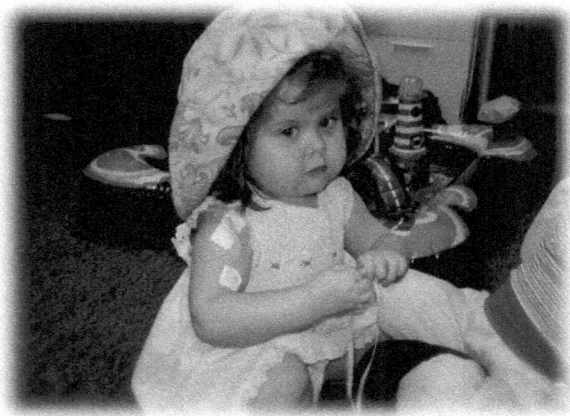

Audrey enjoyed visits to Kathy's "store" in her office.

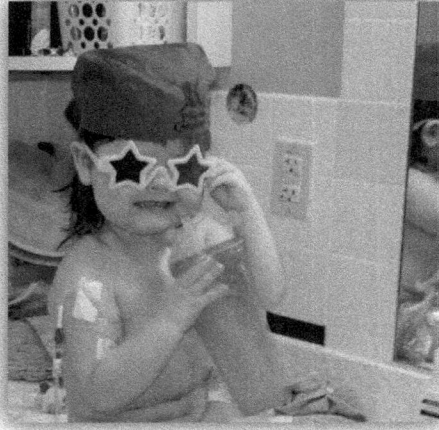

Chapter 2

Clinging to "Normal"

*"We tried to live in the moment and not put our lives on hold . . .
picnics by the river in the lobby and family movie nights."*

As you are reading these pages, you may be new to the whole hospital experience - maybe at the stage of adjusting to your new routine or frankly still dealing with the shock of your child's condition or prognosis. You may never have spent much time, *if any*, in a medical facility.

I remember meeting our NICU neighbors the day after Audrey was born. Their baby's room was decorated like a nursery, and the mom commanded the presence of a veteran. She had her daily routine down to a science, and she appeared to have been there for a while. In fact, I soon learned that her baby had been a NICU resident for three months already. I was amazed! Imagine, three months inpatient and counting!

The day we parted ways as they headed home, I would have been grateful for only three months! I quickly came to realize that *we* would also be there for a while, so I reluctantly moved in. I *kind of* decorated Audrey's first corner, then her next couple of rooms looked almost like home. I set up a little office, and made myself at home in a consultation room adjoining the unit *(when it wasn't in use!)*. There I made phone calls and took care of any business while Audrey was napping or playing with her nurses.

Managing Your Schedule –
(Around countless other schedules!)

A few months into our NICU stay, Kathy, the developmental specialist, helped me set up a schedule for Audrey that the nurses were firmly expected to abide by...*(no more midnight social gatherings at the nurses' station!)* Needless to say, to this day our daughter is always looking for a party!

As Audrey got older and we made return trips to the hospital for extended stays, I still held us to a schedule as much as I could. Cares had to be completed before her set bedtime, and then no unnecessary disruptions after that. There were to be no routine early morning disruptions either, until Audrey was awake; this included intrusions of medical residents and students! When Audrey spent "seasons" *(literally!)* in the hospital, we just had to do what we could to provide her a normal sleep pattern and daily schedule that she could count on.

We had a schedule during the day of when we would have baths and naps, activity times and play times. Another aspect of routine was to surround Audrey with familiar things from home - a favorite stuffed animal or doll, her "blankie", a favorite book or two, and some of her toys.

I made my daily "to do" list as well: phone calls to make, paperwork to complete, shopping and errands to run. I set up babysitting times with volunteers or nurses. I was not able to put life on hold for months at a time. There was still laundry to do, a house that needed cleaned, a yard that needed maintained, and meals that needed to be shopped for and prepared. I made most of our meals at home a few afternoons each week and brought them to the hospital. Our bathroom doubled as a kitchenette. And thankfully during most of our stays, we were in a hospital that housed mini refrigerators in the rooms. I even made fresh-squeezed limeade one summer afternoon – just for fun! The aroma filled the room – a welcome change!

The Value of Sticking to a Routine –

Routine helped each of us adapt to yet another extended hospital stay, and allowed for a smoother adjustment from home to hospital and from hospital back to home. This was key for us because this regimen happened so frequently over the course of five years. I really think it helped our daughter to cope with such major changes, because those changes happened within the confines of something familiar.

Of course, routines were for typical days when Audrey was feeling well and her care was in a "holding pattern". Post-surgery days and more critical stages of her medical history were different. Sometimes these periods came unexpectedly and we had to switch gears to accommodate a *new* routine. Flexibility enabled us to respond to each new challenge rather than just react.

Preserving some of the routine you are used to at home will play a major role in how you are able to deal with such a life change. It will give you a sense of direction midst the confusion, and some personal control midst a situation that is *out* of your control.

Try to hold to aspects of your *personal* routine also as much as possible - a morning walk, albeit in the hallways; your normal diet; continuing with personal or professional business and contacts - to some extent anyway; sending cards or emails; etc. When stuck in a hospital room day after day, it is very easy to whittle away your time in unproductive manners - the tendency may be to just plug in movie after movie for your child, and get stuck in a funk. Your child gets bored; you may find yourself depressed, with time on your hands for every worry and angst. Have a project to put your head or your hands to use - a project for you, projects for your child, and projects for the two of you to do together!

If you live in town, it might do you good to get away and get some laundry taken care of or straighten up a room - to maintain some order in your own home, or unwind in your garden for thirty minutes, pulling weeds. Focusing on something that I *could* control helped me to balance out the areas over which I had absolutely *no* control. It also helped me to have some sense of order in my schedule and in my life. I could still take care of some things that were important to me, and it helped me to feel like I was doing something for my family, too - keeping up our home.

There were also no staff members waltzing into my house like it was their own - *I had privacy!* In fact, I went home a few times to break down emotionally. Living in a fish bowl doesn't lend itself to much privacy. When you need to have a good cry or to be alone for a few moments, a public environment just doesn't cut it!

For those of you who are from out of town, take breaks when you can and find a quiet spot to read, or visit a local park or museum, coffee shop or sporting goods store! Take time to go get your hair done - a little pampering will help you to relax and make you feel better. If your other children come for a visit, this is a great time to take them on an adventure to see something new!

Guest services at your hospital can provide you with some great tips, and may even keep a supply of free passes to local attractions - so make contact with them! Ask the nurses for ideas, too.

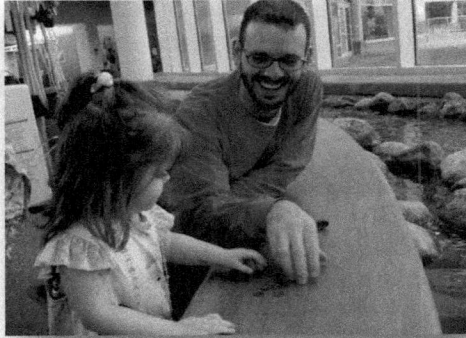

"Penny Flicking" lessons from Dad.

Redefining "Normal" for A While!

We still took time to enjoy things we would have done at home or elsewhere if we weren't cooped up in a hospital. And we adapted activities to fit within our new situation and surroundings. I kept craft supplies on hand - I brought a plastic container with drawers to organize office and craft supplies, i.e. pens, pencils, scissors, note pads, paper clips, thank you notes, glue, stickers, pipe cleaners, etc. We also brought lots of reading, activity, and schoolbooks from home.

Here are a few activities we enjoyed apart from the everyday routine:

- One fall we borrowed the playroom's kitchen - the *real* one - and made apple cobbler for the nurses.
- Audrey's dad taught her how to flick pennies off her thumb and into the "river" in the Children's Hospital lobby.
- I created a Dora clue hunt for Audrey that took us all over the hospital on an adventure, visiting her friends in several offices where she collected her clues- the staff was great to play along!
- We often had Sunday school lessons down by the river in the lobby.
- Audrey's first year of life was documented by photos that I took, since I wasn't able to take her to a studio. I brought props from home; the nurses helped me fix her hair, hold her in a pose, and make faces to get her to smile. We ended up with some pretty good shots!
- My hairdresser, Marie, made "house calls," and came to the hospital to cut Audrey's hair!
- We celebrated the Fourth of July (twice), birthday parties (three of hers, four of mine, two of her dad's), her first Thanksgiving, Christmas, and New Year, along with two Valentine's Days all in the hospital *(not to mention most of our anniversaries!)*.
- Our friend Kathy gave her a little inflatable swimming pool that she played with in her room and outside on the sidewalk *(we transported water in portable urinals!)*. I also got her a little bucket of craft sand, a scoop and shovel, and we would go outside and have little beach parties!
- We were given permission for Audrey to keep a couple of caterpillars in her room that our friend Julie brought to her. She was able to experience the excitement of watching them form a chrysalis and transform into butterflies, then releasing them into the hospital's flower garden.

We went on an adventure everyday when we could. When she couldn't walk, we packed up a wagon and went on our way. I got pretty proficient at manhandling a wagon along with an IV pole!

After six or nine months in the hospital, you *have* to get creative, making the most of your situation, or waste a lot of energy on worry and complaining, making life miserable for yourself and everyone else in close proximity! When I remember our extended hospital stays, many of them bring back some fond memories - the fun things we thought to do, like the wheel chair races her dad would take her on; and the relationships we built with the staff who became our family!

Audrey needed these reprieves, and so did we; and so did the staff. They witness much sadness and grief on a regular basis in their line of work; it does them good to experience happy moments along with the families, too!

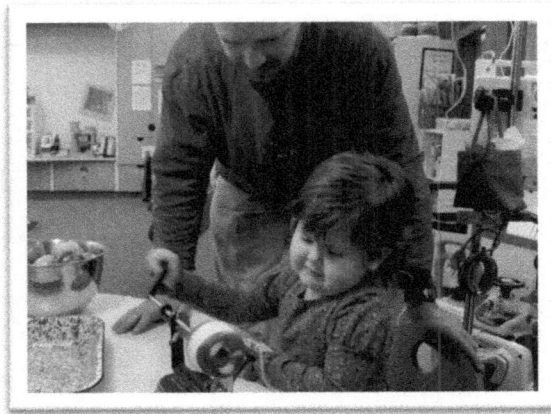

Making apple cobbler for her nurses!

JSYK

"Just so you know..."

You are entering a new phase of "normal" for at least a period of time. Make concessions for it, allowing yourself to be flexible and adaptable when necessary. But embrace some of your familiar routines and schedules when and where you can. This will help your entire family adjust more easily to the changes that are affecting you all.

What are some aspects of your personal and family routines that are important for you to preserve while your loved one is in the hospital?

_____

_____

_____

_____

_____

_____

_____

_____

What challenges are making this difficult for you? Are there issues you need to discuss with someone on the nursing or medical staff, making it easier for you to maintain certain elements of your routine?

_____

_____

_____

_____

_____

_____

_____

_____

_____

_____

_____

_____

_____

_____

_____

_____

_____

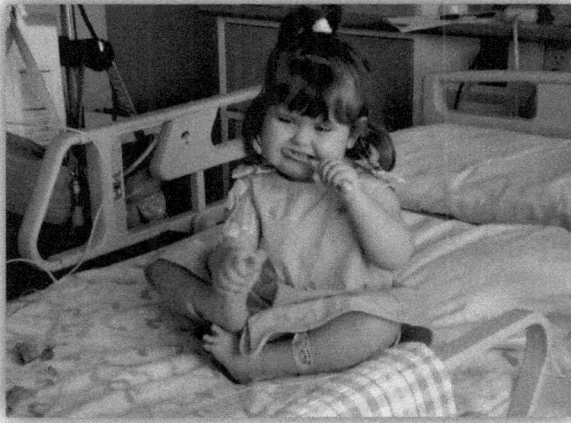

Chapter 3

Home Away From Home

"We came to regard the 5th floor as our vacation home!"

𝒲ℯ frequented Children's Hospital in Omaha to the point that upon arrival, the staff welcomed us like family, and did what they could to give us the best room available! I kept a tally of the rooms we had stayed in. By the end of our stays, we had been in almost all of the twenty-some rooms on 5th floor at some point. We had our favorite rooms - we knew which ones were the quietest and had the best view. We didn't like the rooms right by the exits or pharmacy drops!

The focus in this chapter is on *"creature comforts"*, duly titled by me! I have listed the comforts of home that had a designated spot in our bags. I also prioritized ours according to length of stay. These *"don't leave home without it"* items may offer you some ideas, should you have frequent admissions, also.

Three Days or Less

For Audrey:
- ✓ *Blankie and stuffed animal of choice*
- ✓ *Her favorite cup*
- ✓ *Med list (always keep this in your purse/wallet)*
- ✓ *A few favorite books and movies*
- ✓ *Activities in a small backpack – a few toys and activity/coloring books*
- ✓ *Slip-on shoes or slippers*

For me:
- ✓ *Journal, Bible, and a favorite magazine and book*
- ✓ *Planner or "to do" notebook*
- ✓ *Phone charger*
- ✓ *Laptop (I didn't have one for the first few years.)*
- ✓ *Slip-on shoes*

Let your child pack as much of his own things as he can; of course, our lists were for a two to five year old!

A Week or Longer

- ✓ *Audrey's pillow and blanket*
- ✓ *White noise machine*
- ✓ *Personal towels and washcloths for both of us (much softer and better smelling!)*
- ✓ *Extra money tucked away for meals, snacks, coffee, trip to the gift shop, etc.*
- ✓ *Folder for paperwork, handouts, business cards of doctors and specialists*
- ✓ *Camera*

An Indefinite Stay –
(Longer than a week or month... or season ... or so!)

- ✓ *All of the above*
- ✓ *Lemon juice to spritz my water (It doubles as a fruit & veggie wash!)*
- ✓ *A favorite mug and drinking glass*
- ✓ *Vase with fresh flowers (During a summer stay, I would bring cuttings from my own flower garden.)*
- ✓ *My own pillow and blanket, our own sheets (For hospital beds, dorm-sized sheets work best; I just used a top sheet on the couch and doubled it over.)*
- ✓ *A couple of small baskets to store things, i.e. extra plastic tableware, condiments, snacks, books and toys, or odds & ends and office supplies.*
- ✓ *Office supplies included: note paper, sticky notes, pens & pencils, sharpie, scissors, mini stapler, paper clips, thank you notes, batteries, small screwdriver for battery operated toys.*
- ✓ *I also had a portable file tote with me for storing paperwork.*
- ✓ *Small reading lamp (This was great for use when Audrey was sleeping.)*

When we couldn't be home, we brought a little "home" with us for each stay. It also helped for our hospital room to be clean and comfortable, and neat and tidy. The room felt more inviting and personal when it reflected a little of us. I would arrange Audrey's toys and books to create a little girl's world. In my corner, I set my books and magazines and other items in a nice presentation - it brought me a bit of peace!

As I review this chapter, I realize some readers may see these comments as "trite", but when a patient and his family are literally *living* at the hospital, these details make all the difference. Trust me, you will feel more comfortable, more relaxed.

If you are a "germaphobe" like me, then bring your own cleaning wipes. I did, and I wiped down all surfaces, just to feel more at ease. Do what makes you comfortable! When I or anyone else would enter the room, it felt like a bedroom or studio apartment instead of a sterile, bare hospital ward. Pleasant and familiar surroundings helped us feel more at home, which was important since it *was* our home for so much of the time!

JSYK

"Just so you know..."

If you make your child's hospital room a little like home and create pleasant surroundings, you will lift *everyone's* mood! It will promote good emotional health for your child *and* you, along with the rest of the family. You'll be providing a "healing environment."

Jot down some things you or your child would like to have while at the hospital to make your stay a little more comfortable ...

_____

_____

_____

_____

_____

_____

_____

_____

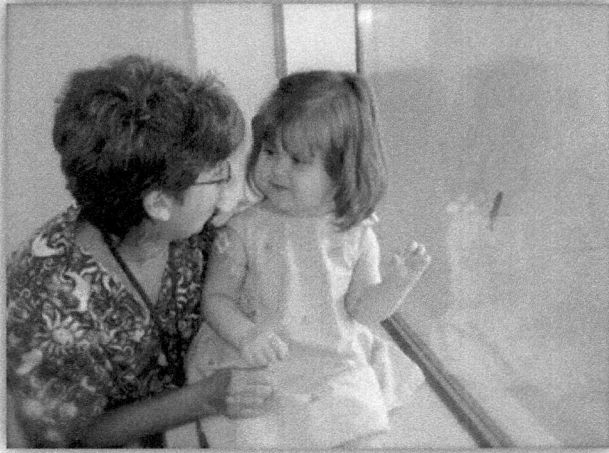

Chapter 4

Keeping your Outlook in Check

"It was our lot, we came to accept it, and we made the best of it."

On a Positive Note...
(Perks to prize-winning "frequent admit" status)

- Consider your savings on all of the toilet paper, utilities, soap, diapers, and coffee provided!
- Free housekeeping at your disposal!
- Free babysitting if you and your spouse need a night out!
- All the new friends you make in the staff and other *"in"*mates, if you will ... sometimes it's like a family reunion!
- A room with a view *(hopefully)*!
- A lifetime supply of scissors!
- Our very own "Prox" card and armband, allowing us "privileged access!"
- A "state-of-the-art" playroom!

- If new admit rooms are stocked with little stuffed bears, your gift dilemma is solved for a while - cousins and friends all get a hospital souvenir for their birthdays!
- Free and unlimited movies!
- Your toddler may develop an impressive vocabulary and understanding of terms like the following: *"occlusion," "blood pressure cuff," "tegaderm," "steri-strips," "opmy* (ostomy) bag, *"hook up to suction," "NG tube," "G-button," "TPN," "HIJK"* (which means EKG to a three year old!).

Roll with the Punches!

Maintaining a sense of humor always helps in a tense situation. Being adaptable also allowed us to continue in a state of mind to make appropriate decisions for our daughter's care, address the medical staff with the right questions, and stay on top of what was happening to our child. We also held to the opinion that the medical staff knew what was best for Audrey. However, we also developed a confidence and rapport with them to challenge a decision or offer an alternative solution.

Faith: Maintaining Hope...

I firmly believe that the Lord's grace and the prayers of hundreds of people being lifted up on our family's behalf carried us through. For us, God was our stronghold. And our faith that God had a plan, and that He was truly working through our circumstances and carrying us through gave us hope to keep our sights above what was happening to Audrey in the near and present. This truth distanced us from despair.

Gratitude and Searching out the Good-

Think of specific benefits and blessings in your life. Some may be within your circumstances while others are in spite of your circumstances. Here were a few for us:

Locale -

Thankfully, for us, we lived less than ten minutes away from the two hospitals where our daughter would receive care. In fact, we relocated to Omaha just before we learned I was pregnant. Little did we know at the time the medical needs our daughter would have, that would be met specifically by the best qualified staff we could find - right at our doorstep!

Top-notch Staff and Facilities -

Patients of Children's Hospital came from all over the country for care from the wonderful doctors available. And The Nebraska Medical Center was world renown for its transplant program, which would ultimately save Audrey's life.

Timing of Transplant -

When the unimaginable occurred, being listed for a transplant, Audrey was in overall good health for transplant status, despite her failing organs. Also, her amazing team of doctors up to that point had kept her organs healthy long enough for her body to grow and develop, and for the transplant program to progress and improve before she would become a recipient.

Finances-

Financial coverage was thankfully already in place. Audrey had long exceeded the maximum coverage allowed on our family's insurance plan; however, she had qualified for Medicaid, given her specific medical needs.

Support-

We had a local support system in place - wonderful friends and church family, as well as family members who were able to travel to be there as needed.

Journaling-

There are abundant benefits to journaling. It helps you to keep track of information and events. It's a way to sort out your thoughts and emotions. It can serve as a way to problem-solve and to think of questions you need to ask. As you note the answers to those questions, you have them to refer to later on, if need be. Journaling always helped me unwind and unload from the challenges of the day and to regain perspective. It was a *great* venue for keeping my outlook in check!

I encourage you just to start at whatever point you are. You can use a simple spiral notebook - a size that is comfortable for you. There is no need to feel the pressure to journal everyday. I sure didn't. You have enough pressure, right now. Just write as you have the opportunity. Keep your journal with you as much as you can, so that when you have a few minutes, you can take advantage and jot down some thoughts.

During our first hospital stay of nine months, I didn't journal a thought. I did well to make it through a day and not lose my mind. By the time we returned, I was ready - and I had a lot of catching up to do! I began with the circumstances of the moment, and then I set aside a section of my journal to work on past events. I recommend starting sooner than later. I have forgotten much of those first several months.

I also suggest that you divide your journal into themes. If your notebook doesn't have separate sections, then use post-it notes for markers - borrow some from the nurse's station! These are the sections I have included in my journals:

- Gratitude and blessings: Try daily to note something you are thankful for, or something positive that has happened.
- Funny moments and humorous quips people say *(especially your child - to add to her baby book or whatever mementos you keep at home)*.
- Random thoughts, events, and emotions.
- Questions for concerned parties, troubleshooting ideas and solutions.
- Spiritual insight, scripture, and quotes filled with encouragement and wisdom, along with life lessons being learned.
- Inspirations and ideas for improving your situation and those of other families; thoughts to pass along to hospital staff and executives as well as home healthcare staff.

You might want to record the following in a separate notebook. They were sure helpful to me:

- Visitor list - you could invite visitors to sign their name in a notebook and add a comment if they wish; they might just leave you a thought that could help you through some difficult days ahead. They also offer a nostalgic element to return to and read again a few years down the road.
- A list of gifts received; it can double as a thank-you note list.

As I was writing this book, I came across a journal entry I had made at a conference workshop sponsored by the hospital. At the time Audrey was inpatient, and had been for about four months. The workshop leader suggested journaling observations about your child that you might forget later. (This reminded me of my dad, who filmed "miles" of footage of Audrey while she was in the NICU, in case she never made it home.) Later in my journal, I wrote down several observations I remembered about Audrey that very day - she was about three and a half at the time. And I am so glad I took the time to jot those moments down; they are priceless to go back and pore over. If I hadn't written them down, I wouldn't have those memories today - they were long forgotten! I'd like to share them with you, because they make such a powerful point all by themselves!

- Her upbeat spirit when I returned this afternoon
- The dolly's shoe she was fixated on in the playroom
- The way she'd swing her arms and jump in the hallway - calling them her "exercises!"
- Her eagerness for her medicine
- Calling out to Debbie for stickers when we headed into the hallway tonight
- Pushing her hair away from her eyes

The workshop leader stressed the value of writing about important events in life, both tragic *and* happy.   She said that it helps the immune system - it can therapeutic, a part of self-care. It acts as a release for pent-up emotions.

She also had us list our worries and anxieties of the moment. It helps me to go back and review what I wrote four years earlier. I didn't even remember doing this exercise - I had not read these journal entries since that day in the workshop! The following is what I listed:

- Audrey's existing condition
- Her insurance situation *(She had recently maxed out her insurance coverage! Yikes!!)*
- Paperwork looming over my head
- The stress of finances

- Relationship with my husband
- Schedule
- Lack of good sleep
- Fear of continued complications with Audrey's health - scar tissue, fistulas, more surgeries, X-rays, IV lines, meds, condition of veins

Hopefully, sharing a few ideas of mine will help you appreciate the value of journaling. Consider trying it for yourself!

Control-

When you find yourself in a situation that is out of your control, it is important to identify and take possession of what is *in* your control. This can allow you to "rein in" your despairing thoughts and manage your outlook more effectively.

We were unable to heal our daughter - we had to totally rely on medical professionals and God's providence. The doctors and their staff had the training and expertise to do amazing things to help our daughter's prognosis.

The Lord had His hand in every aspect of her destiny - leading us to Omaha and the tremendous medical teams awaiting us; guiding the doctors' decisions and hands in the operating room; having the entire design of Audrey's life in His plan, from start to finish; as well as how He would use this experience in our own lives to form and strengthen us. Believing this was vital when we found ourselves watching from the sidelines, unable to do a thing for our daughter.

In terms of Audrey's care, it helped to be attentive to her daily needs - physical and emotional. We *could* be in charge of many elements, i.e. cuing the nurses on the best way to approach Audrey and the best time to do her daily assessment. We *could* be hands on in her care - helping with baths and with wound dressing changes, ostomy care, and administration of her medications.

We could *not* change the fact that our daughter would likely need a small bowel transplant. However, we *could* take control of her care post-transplant. We could be diligent with her medications and her nutrition; her overall health and well-being; her development and coping skills; her education, along with the nurturing, love, and guidance that would help her to thrive. Taking ownership of our daughter's care in the areas that we *could* sure made a difference in how *"in"* or *"out"* of control we felt. It helped us to have a better grip when the situation demanded that someone else call the shots, while we stood by as spectators!

When in the hospital, we had little control over *several* aspects of life - in certain areas of Audrey's care, in her schedule and *our* schedule, our room and privacy...But we *could* coordinate with the staff and arrange a suitable routine and schedule that would work for both them and us. We *could* make requests regarding some elements of her care. We *could* simply put up a *"do not disturb"* sign on our door, understanding that it would not always be acknowledged. We *could* request adequate notice on all procedures so that we could plan accordingly. We *could* arrange someone to sit with Audrey while we tended to other matters, including ourselves and our marriage. We *did* plan an occasional date!

Emotionally we *could* control how we interacted with the staff when there was a disagreeable issue, how we would respond to unwanted disruptions, our overall attitude day in and day out with our circumstances. Sometimes this meant stepping back and taking a deep breath before reacting! We had the choice to interject humor when possible and to expose Audrey to fun activities throughout the day to keep the mood upbeat around her.

I made a journal entry early on which sums up the dilemma of parents when they are not the only one in charge of their child:

> *"When you spend a few weeks or longer in the hospital,*
> *or anywhere for that matter, you begin to mentally take*
> *up residence...*

*I have found that I get into a system - my "hospital"
routine. This means there are certain times when we
schedule things, slots when I fit in meals or my "to-do"
list... our schedules must work around doctors' visits or
rounds, administration of meds or other needed cares,
when the dogs are coming for a visit, or when the "girls"
(teen volunteers) are here to play.*

*Part of this rigor is the phenomenon of "shared
custody" of your child's care. Who calls the shots? Do
you give your child a bath or does the nursing staff give
the bath - is it on your timeline or theirs? What do you
have to ask permission to do, concerning her care?"*

This was a disheartening reality from the day Audrey was born.
As soon as she was delivered, the hospital took ownership of her. I
was allowed to see her for a couple of seconds, and then they carried
her off to prepare her for surgery. We were not solely in charge of her
until they released her from the hospital almost nine and a half
months later!

I remember the first time Dallas asked me if I had washed
Audrey's face. She was maybe a few weeks old, and he noticed some
"crusties" on her face. The thought had not even occurred to me to
wash her face. I was barely allowed to hold her at the time. If we
wanted to hold her, we had to ask for permission and get the nurse's
assistance. Audrey was dressed in tubes and lines that were
precariously place all *over* and *in* her fragile and tiny body. She had
to be handled with extreme care. In all reality, I was probably afraid
to wash her face - afraid I would hurt her or tug on a line, or worse
yet, that I was infringing on the duty of the nurses!

During the very brief period that Audrey was being bottle-fed,
nurses might determine her feeding schedule for the day, based on

the schedule of their other patients - without consulting me, her mother. This would change from day to day; I couldn't even make my own feeding schedule for *my* baby! I thought it was outrageous!! So I had to adjust my schedule everyday to accommodate the nurse's schedule. It really upset me! I should have been more assertive about reconciling the situation. The nurses had multiple feeding and care schedules to juggle with their different patients, and they didn't realize how this affected my feelings as a parent.

Confront-

I was in a new role ... this was my *first* child and my *first* experience with a child as a hospital patient. I thought the medical staff had the final say in every aspect, and that they were not to be questioned. I have long since abandoned that theory – emerging with a whole new personality! By the time we passed the baton on to other parents, and said "adios" to our clinical way of life, *we* were instructing the *staff* on how to care for our child! I had become the lioness protecting her cub, *"and don't you dare mess with me!"*

Audrey required such intensive and specialized care in the beginning that I felt like a spectator, *not* her mother. Actually, when I think about it, I was more of a "Nurse in Training!" This was not an error of the hospital. I feel, however, that if the hospital staff were more aware of the parents' awkward position, perhaps parenting and caregiving from the staff could be a more efficient and effective team effort! Maybe the discharge staff and social worker could intervene early on to help define more clearly the role of the parent for the sake of *all* parties involved during the family's hospital stay - no matter how long it will be.

JSYK

"Just so you know..."

The more you step up and confront your situation, the better you will be able to deal with the hardships - both present and those to come.

Confront with gratitude: What is something good that happened today?

_____

_____

_____

_____

Confront by journaling your thoughts: What are you struggling with? What questions or concerns would you like to address with your child's care team?

_____

_____

_____

_____

_____

_____

Confront what is out of your control by identifying what is in your control! What issues are difficult for you to accept right now? What is making you feel out of control in your present circumstances?

_____

_____

_____

_____

_____

_____

_____

_____

_____

Where or how can you contribute, concerning your child's condition and care? How can these steps give you more control in your circumstances?

_____

_____

_____

_____

_____

_____

_____

_____

_____

_____

_____

_____

_____

_____

_____

_____

_____

_____

_____

_____

P.S.

As I was completing this book, our family was confronted with some new challenges, testing my "outlook" and faith! So I started an experiment this morning, that I plan to carry out on a regular daily basis for awhile. Late last night, I was feeling down, worried, agitated, annoyed, *angry* about multiple issues that seemed to be escalating in my life, our lives. I had to come to terms with the reality that these problems weren't affecting only me but our family, as well. So first, I took the focus off of just myself. I then realized that I was frowning. I was reminded of how often my daughter asks me what I'm mad about; when I ask her what she means, she comments that she can see it on my face - and I then notice that my brows are furrowed, and I probably am frowning, not smiling. She can tell when something is wrong and I am deep in thought ... more likely deep in *worry*!

I extended myself a personal challenge: To smile! It is quite an effort to smile naturally when you are upset! However, I purposely smiled, and without exaggerating, I immediately felt better! - *Then I shook a few dark chocolate chips into my mouth for good measure, and that, of course, gave a little boost to the effect!* - But in all seriousness, I was amazed at how little I really smile; especially, when I am alone, and anxious about something. I tend to worry, when my mind is not otherwise occupied, and when I am not purposing to be thankful!

Today, news and circumstances only got worse - I was struggling not to feel hopeless, and I remembered my challenge - to smile! I formed my troubled face into a smile several times throughout the day with the same result - an instant lift in my countenance! It didn't solve my problems, but it did help with my outlook, to remember to be thankful, and to be hopeful that there is a solution; I just need to take the *next right step!!* I have given that step some thought, and now have a plan of action!

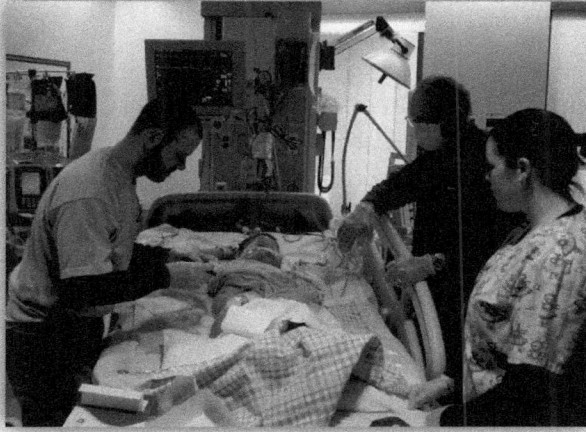

Chapter 5

Be Proactive and Involved!

"When you find yourself in a situation that is out of your control, it is important to identify and take possession of what is in your control."
(Carrying on from Chapter 4!)

*T*he more *proactive* and *involved* you are with your child's care the more *control* you will have in your situation. You will have a better sense of your child's condition and a more complete understanding of how to deal with challenges that arise. You will be better prepared to ask the right questions, and more equipped to handle your child's care at home, if need be.

Active Player Status on the Team ...

The role you play on your child's care team is just as important as that of any staff member. You know your child, and you can read most of his signs better than any medical professional. The more you participate, the better the care your child will receive. It will also help you to feel more involved in the situation, giving you a greater sense of control and purpose, as I just mentioned in the last chapter.

You also hold the unique position of overseeing the care your child receives from each doctor or specialist. It might be you who opens communication amongst the different areas of expertise, encouraging teamwork. In some hospitals, the staff from these different areas may already work closely together, developing integral care plans for their patients, as each expert offers his or her perspective to the plan. However, if you don't think this is happening, or if you notice something that hasn't been considered in the plan, then bring it to the table.

The more you understand what is involved in your child's care, the more you will be able to foster this teamwork and communication amongst all the schools of thought being offered. For example, GI (Gastroenterology) and Cardiology may have differing opinions on when it is appropriate to start feeding a patient who has undergone heart surgery. A physical therapist may have to communicate closely with a surgeon, as she is working with a post-surgery patient. This will ensure she is posing just the right amount of challenge to her patient without hindering healing. A nutritionist, rather than a surgeon, may be the better party to consult for healthy menu options for your child.

It's really important for you to be keenly aware of how your child is feeling - physically, emotionally, and mentally; how he looks, any indication that something is not right. You will likely notice red flags before anyone else. Trust your intuition, and be confident in vocalizing it; *you* are your child's voice to the hospital staff. An example of this from experience concerns Audrey's body temperature. Her normal body temperature tends to run a little low.

If I recognized her temperature climbing above normal, I knew to keep an eye on it. Once it climbed above ninety-nine degrees, I knew we might have an issue, and advised her nurse so that she could keep close tabs on it. We learned how to use the hospital thermometers, so we could take her temperature whenever we felt we needed to.

We also involved ourselves in about every aspect of her care, such as changing her ostomy bag, managing various tubes that were hooked up to suction or that needed flushed. As parents, we could help maintain consistency in her care, because we were there day in and day out, and were present if there was a change in care. If a new nurse on shift had a question on how exactly to perform a certain care, we would be able to step in and lend a hand. I have also learned that information can get misconstrued, misunderstood, or overlooked all together as it is passed from one nurse to another and to another, as the shifts change and the days pass - much like the telephone game!

My appreciation runs deep for the team of doctors, nurses, and specialists that cared for Audrey. I felt like they really had our backs - especially the nurses and pediatric surgical team at Children's Hospital. We could address any concern with them, and they never made us feel as though we were a nuisance or over-reacting to a situation. They always listened to us, and even respected us enough to run a plan by us before carrying it out, to make sure we approved. I think that the mutual rapport and trust between us came from several years of working together so closely for our daughter's cause.

JSYK

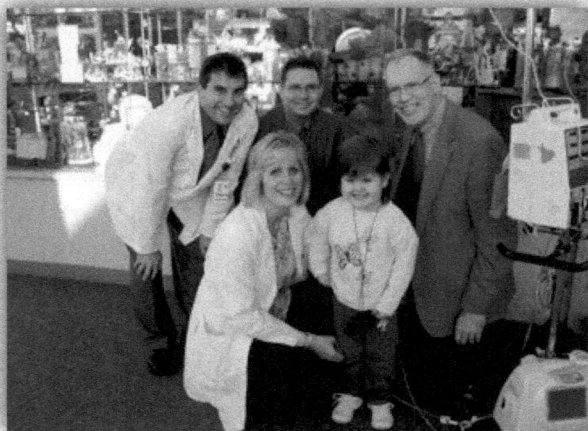

*We couldn't have chosen a better team if we had to. It was an
honor to work with the surgical staff at Children's Hospital in
Omaha. They became like family. And Dr. Raynor credits
Audrey to adding a few gray hairs to his head!*

Be in the Know ... and just Ask!

Request a copy of your child's care plan, so that you know the
schedule of cares and administration of medicines. This will help
you in planning your child's personal schedule, as well as yours. It is
equally important for you, as the consistent caregiver, to review how
certain cares are completed, so if you see a discrepancy in the care
plan, you can address it. For example, many times I noticed that a
certain care procedure had not recently been updated in the care
plan. So if a new nurse was on duty for a shift and wasn't aware of
the change, she would just follow the care plan as it was written. If

you notice an error or an omission, bring it to the staff's attention so unnecessary mistakes may be prevented.

Ask to be kept informed of the schedule for lab work and X-rays, other procedures and tests, so that you can know ahead of time to prepare and plan *your* schedule. There was nothing more aggravating than having a staff member from radiology show up at 7:00 in the morning - *without warning* - to take Audrey downstairs for a test. Neither of us would be ready, we would have to scramble around getting dressed, getting tubes and lines unhooked, and I wouldn't have had my morning coffee yet! *Now how bad is that?!* Well, you get the picture; after so many months of other people determining your daily schedule, you reach a point when you just get mad, and your tolerance level drops to an all time low!

Another example is that if a trip to radiology is scheduled, ask about the plan if they haven't yet revealed it to you. If there are orders to complete a barium study, you may be there for a few hours. This would be important information to know. We didn't always know! Maybe I was expecting a 20 minute trip downstairs for a quick X-ray, planning to catch breakfast after we returned, only to find out - *once we arrived* – that this would be a barium study, and that multiple X-rays were required, as the contrast traveled through the digestive system. We would be there for two or three hours with nothing to eat, and Audrey having nothing to do... Don't be afraid to ask!

At the same time, try to be considerate of the staff's schedule and tasks they must tend to while on shift. Overall, the majority of the staff members are trying to do their best for your child's benefit and for yours. You probably have already experienced nurses going out of their way to do something extra special for your child, or taking the time to exercise extreme care when it is important. They may have even offered to sit with your child, insisting that you go catch a meal or a rest.

To make things flow the best for your family and for other families, as well as the staff, start taking note of schedules - shift changes and report times, lunch and break times. This way, if you need something from your nurse or other staff members, you can make those requests when they are free to accommodate you. Learn who the other nurses are in the unit, and who the care partners, techs or nurse's assistants are. It will make it easier and quicker for you to determine what requests to make of whom! If you become the one primarily in charge of certain aspects of your child's care, such as bath time or changing linens, you may be able to learn where supplies are kept and how to access them.

This makes it much easier to retrieve or request something you need if perhaps your nurse isn't available - it allows you more independence and convenience; you don't have to wait around for more towels if no one is available to assist you. If you are like me, it may also make you feel better about not hassling your nurse all the time for trivial things, such as sheets or a washcloth! Ask to help administer your child's meds, so that you are accustomed to the method and schedule, should she need to continue her meds at home.

Your position also involves asking questions - this is a right, a privilege, and an obligation. No question is inconsequential; *every* question is important, if it means you understanding your child's prognosis, his care, and the reason behind anything a staff member does or proposes to do. Without realizing it, medical personnel tend to communicate with individuals outside the clinical world with the same "shop talk" or medical jargon that they use with their colleagues. Call me ignorant, but I didn't understand the word *"distended"* prior to Audrey's admittance in the NICU! And I didn't know what a "sat probe" was for - for oxygen saturation, *of course!* What does *that* mean*??!! Other* parents have understood the term "room air" to be of French origin (*It does have a certain French flair when it rolls off your tongue!*).

Just ask - it beats remaining in the dark! You will neither be the first *nor* the last parent to ask for clarification of a term that seems to run fluent amongst the nurses and other medical staff!

Request test results, such as from lab draws and X-rays. Often times, the results are available and never passed on to the parent or patient unless they ask. Find out your child's normal vitals range: normal heartbeat, oxygen saturation level, blood pressure, etc. As you view the monitors your child is hooked up to, you can observe whether a number is abnormal and ask the nurse about it.

As I will address later on, many of these numbers are indicators of whether there are specific issues going on with the patient, such as pain and discomfort, or not enough oxygen in the blood. Know your child's blood type, as well, and record it with other vital information about your child. Request to sit in on the nurses' report. This is the "briefing" at shift change that takes place between the current nurse and the nurse who is beginning the next shift. This is the most excellent way for you as the parent to hear firsthand what exactly transpired during the last shift, and the care plan for the shift to come. Test results are revealed, any changes to your child's care plan, such as with medications or new procedures, dressings, etc. And if something is reported wrongly or omitted, you can make a correction. If changes are made, it would be good for you to review the care plan for the following shift and sit in on report in order to verify that the correction was made in your child's care plan. If you go home for the night, it's okay to call the night nurse to check in on your child. And if you can't be there for report at the end of her shift, call before shift change and ask for a report over the phone.

You might also find it helpful, for future reference, to take notes during report on changes that are being made, and to write down answers you receive from conversations with the doctors. These notes can be invaluable tools when the time comes to explain things to someone else! I would consult with Audrey's medical team in the morning, and by that evening I would be capable of relaying *maybe* fifty percent of the information to my husband or to others who called for an update! It was difficult to remember everything if I didn't take notes; and I didn't always pass along explanations as thoroughly and as accurately as the doctors had communicated things to me. By the time Audrey had her transplant, we owned a laptop computer; and shortly after the doctors' rounds, I would try and take a few moments to send a detailed update to my dad, who then passed along the information to hundreds of our supporters through email or our Carepage. This method was much more effective in preserving the majority of the conversation I had just had with the transplant team! My brother, Brad, was in the hospital recently for a procedure. When the doctor came out of the OR to visit with my sister-in-law, she recorded her conversation with the doctor so that she would remember it in detail to review with Brad later on. I thought this was ingenious! Be sure to ask the doctor's permission first, if you choose this option!

If you better understand concepts with a visual description, draw diagrams or pictures, or ask your child's doctor to do so. This was very beneficial to us. Decide, with someone else's advice, what you should learn about your child's condition and what information you should avoid researching. There is a load of data at our fingertips these days – some of it pertinent, some of it unnecessary. It is important to understand as much as you *need* to, without being aware of *everything*! Any information you research should cover not only your child's condition, but also general good health practices for the affected organs or body parts, so that the care of your child will be optimal.

Be an informed caregiver, and become a proponent in the nutrition and exercise of your child. For example, when a "clear diet" is allowed, limit sugary items in this category such as jello, popsicles, juices and sodas. The doctors may permit them, but consider healthier options, such as clear broths, teas, and ice chips. If your child is bedridden or admitted for an extended hospital stay, I would recommend that some therapy or exercise be part of his care plan. Address any questions or concerns about this with your child's team of doctors.

Tell it Like it is!

In the next chapter, I will be addressing pain management and medications. One important issue I will cover is that of understanding tolerance levels and certain side effects of medications that a patient may display, and how you as the parent are the best source of information on how certain meds may affect your child specifically. This goes along with the use of other medical supplies or procedures that affect your child in certain ways. If your child ends up in a new clinic or hospital somewhere, he is a blank slate until the staff reads his records and receives medical history from his parents or caregiver. For example, if your child reacts badly to a certain adhesive placed on his skin, this information should be posted in his medical history and reviewed with the staff responsible for his care. If he typically has an adverse reaction to a certain pain or anti-anxiety drug, make this known to new attending staff members. If he is going into surgery, be sure to review these reactions with the anesthesiologist who will be caring for your child.

Be persistent if you are not getting the care that you think is needed, the answers you are looking for, or the action that you feel is necessary or best for your child. In the case of your child's well-being, it is better to be *over* cautious than to ignore an instinct you may have about something. There were a few times when we were concerned about Audrey's condition, and didn't feel as though her nurse or other responsible party treated it with the urgency that they should have. So we would take matters into our own hands, whether it was a needed dressing change or a call to the surgeon, or other staff member.

If you *are* worried or there is reason for concern, use discretion on what you reveal to the patient. If it's not necessary to make your child aware of disturbing or frightening news just yet, then wait and don't alarm him unnecessarily. And you may want to advise the medical staff to step outside the room to discuss certain matters that you don't want your child overhearing.

Enough is Enough!

One ongoing issue we had with Audrey was the care of her central line. She had had so many central lines and PICC lines, and she was quickly losing venous *(IV)* access. When she couldn't eat, they were literally her lifelines! We couldn't afford to lose access! But she would get infection after infection, and as we became more informed and more involved, we observed careless practices by some of the nursing staff that very well could have been the source of the infection.

We finally set our own protocol for Audrey's line care. It was the best way to insure minimal risk of infection, when she couldn't afford any more line infections! We set aside a separate box of gloves for line care exclusively. Those gloves could not be accessed without clean hands or for any other care. They were for *Audrey's* protection. The general box of gloves was for the *staff's* protection. We noticed that if a diaper was going to be changed or an ostomy bag emptied, hands weren't necessarily washed just before reaching for gloves. The nurse might then reach into the same box for a pair to access Audrey's central line.

Sometimes before accessing the line, the nurse would lay the gloves on the dirty bed linens, and then put them on without washing her hands. Those gloves would then come into contact with the central line port. It sounds like a great country song, doesn't it: *"Those Gloves!"* Well, we declared war on *those gloves!*

We also requested a *minimum* full 10-second scrub *with friction* on both the outside of the port as well as the end of the port, allowing the area to dry completely. We asked that a mask be worn, as well. We finally requested no students or new nurses access her line. We were desperate to preserve her veins! My philosophy was: "Why take the chance?" With so many risks and consequences to consider, it only made sense to be as cautious as we could!

Because we were *"in"* for such frequent and extended stays, we also maintained a list of nurses that we requested be the only ones to care for Audrey. They were familiar with her condition and with her complex care; and we could trust them to be consistent. These nurses were also the only ones who would do line dressing changes, and they faithfully followed protocol; this greatly put our minds at ease. We welcomed nursing students to observe these fragile cares, but after so many line issues, they were not allowed to touch any access point on her central line.

I share this story with a passion, because central line infections have taken their toll on more health-compromised children. It is so unnecessary when carelessness is the cause of it! When I was expressing my concern about this to a nurse after Audrey's transplant, she promptly informed me with confidence that Audrey *would* get a line infection, simply because she had a compromised immune system. In my opinion, that nurse had already lowered the bar, *inviting* trouble with the line! Please, if you have any concerns about the care of your child, address them with someone of influence. Your child's life, not your reputation as the "difficult parent," is what is at stake! Besides, if you handle the situation firmly yet graciously, the staff will appreciate your assertiveness for your child's sake.

JSYK

The Importance of Safety Protocols ...

If you have any questions about the care being given, don't hesitate to ask *before* something goes wrong! This is especially critical if a particular nurse is new to your child's care. Find out the protocols for your hospital and/or unit: Are your nurses following the proper safety guidelines? Is a floating nurse ever assigned to your child? Floats are nurses who are standing in as a substitute in a different unit due to shortage of staff. Is the float aware of important protocols for that particular unit, especially if they are essential to the care of your child? Standards can vary from one hospital to another or even amongst different units.

An example is that the care of a central line might be different for an adult patient versus a pediatric patient. We experienced this with Audrey her first night or two after transplant. She was assigned a floating nurse who worked with adult patients, not pediatric patients. The protocol for accessing a central line and changing a central line dressing was different than what we had been accustomed to at Children's Hospital. We had to address this issue with the nurse when we saw her not following the proper guidelines for cleaning a central line port. Remind him or her respectfully that it is in the interest of your child that certain standards and protocols be practiced. It might lower your anxiety and eliminate potential awkwardness if you take time to personally review these protocols and your concerns with any new staff at the beginning of a shift, before an issue can even present itself!

Establish high standards to protect both your child and you from nasty germs! Begin with good hand washing – for you, your child, staff that comes into contact with your child, and visitors! Be mindful of contagious symptoms that could be passed to your already health-compromised child.

Require essential staff to wear masks if they display any symptoms; nonessential staff should be kept out of contact with your child if they display any symptoms. Visitors with symptoms should go straight home until they are better! If *you* are feeling sick, then you should stay away from your child, as well! I had more cold sores during Audrey's hospitalizations than any other time in my life, I think! During her first couple of weeks in the NICU, I had to wear a mask, because my upper lip was one big cold sore!

Any staff member will agree that a hospital is an oversized "petri dish" full of active germs that can easily be passed from one room to the other, from one patient to the other through contact from staff members, door handles, cell phones, and shoes! I was always very careful if anything of ours touched the floor. Patients have been known to contract some awful viruses and bacteria from carelessness – a bandage falling to the floor and then being used on the patient, unsafe hand washing before a procedure, careless dressing changes – Audrey included!

Remember Your "Please" and "Thank You"!

Make sure to share your appreciation with everyone involved in the care of your young patient, including the housekeeping team and food services. They work hard for you, and generally go unnoticed. Try to ease their loads a little by keeping your room picked up and a surface cleared for the food tray as your child's meal is delivered. They are just as important to the team as the rest of the members!

Plus, if you are kind and respectful to them, they will likely return the favor, such as honoring your request to not enter the room during inopportune times, nap time or in the middle of the night!

Having Someone in Your Corner –

A friend on the "inside" can carry you far! Seek out a staff member or two with whom you have rapport, whose opinions you trust, and who will go the extra mile for you *and* your child. First, their position may lend credibility and clout that you do not have. They can get things done, and people are likely to listen to them.

Secondly, their expertise can be valuable in problem solving, and they bring a different perspective to the table. They may offer a simple solution to a concern of yours without making a huge issue of it, and with quicker results than if you had tried resolving it alone. Such a liaison can help carry the burden and relieve some of the responsibility you are trying to shoulder by yourself.

This person *or* persons may be able to communicate more effectively to your child's care team something that is bothering you or that you both see as a concern or issue. In a tense situation, they can operate as a neutral party, lending more objectivity to the circumstances and less emotion than you might at the time.

When the time comes to go home, they can help make sure things are in order and that you have the support you need. They are well informed of your child's needs and the level of care that will be required at home. They can go to bat for you, working with the discharge nurses and home health team to address any fears or apprehensions you may have, considering all aspects of assistance that you may need. And make sure their direct phone number is at your fingertips ... Program it into your phone!!

JSYK

"Just so you know..."

Health care personnel can make mistakes. It's the right thing as a parent to require diligence in your child's care. It's okay to question a staff member. If you see someone on the verge of possibly doing something wrong, speak up before it's too late!

How can you start being a more active player on your child's care team?

_____

_____

_____

_____

_____

_____

_____

_____

_____

_____

Are there any areas of concern that need to be addressed right now?

_____

_____

_____

_____

_____

_____

_____

_____

_____

_____

In what areas do you need to become more informed, regarding your child's condition or care?   For example, are you familiar with your child's meds - what they are for, the side affects, the schedule of administration, and how they are administered?

_____

_____

_____

_____

_____

_____

_____

Who could be your point person? Whom do you know and trust to be a liaison for your family? Start thinking of some things they can specifically help you with; allow them to elaborate on what they feel they can do for you!

_____

_____

_____

_____

_____

_____

_____

_____

_____

_____

_____

_____

_____

_____

_____

_____

_____

_____

_____

_____

_____

_____

_____

_____

_____

_____

_____

_____

_____

_____

_____

_____

_____

_____

_____

_____

_____

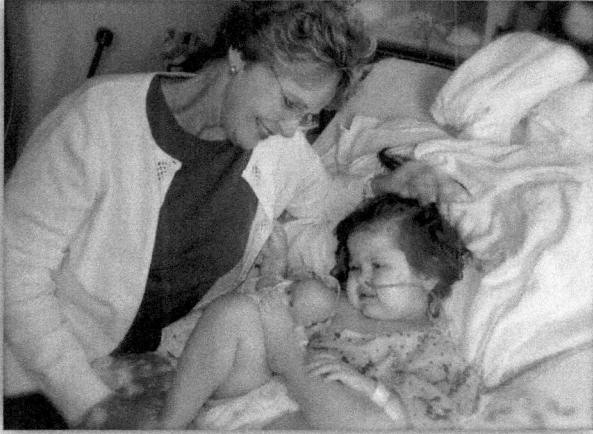

Chapter 6

Pain, Anxiety, Side Effects ... Oh, My!

*"The day Audrey placed a piece of wound vac dressing on my
stomach was a rude awakening to the pain she encountered daily ...
(actually it was the moment I removed the dressing!!)"*

Understanding Pain and Anxiety -

*P*ain is a real and negative force in a patient's recovery and in the overall management of his condition. And though he may be surrounded and supported by empathizers, he really is alone in his discomfort. Unless someone else has been in his position, it is impossible to have a full understanding of the pain and anxiety a patient is experiencing. We as caregivers may be able to sympathize and imagine the pain, but it is never the same as *feeling* the pain.

Anxiety is just as real as pain for these patients undergoing not only unpleasant procedures and clinical experiences, but also facing potentially uncertain futures. Imagine this reality playing itself out in a small child. Add to the equation, the unfamiliar surroundings of a hospital and staff, strangers probing and engaging with him, treatments which may be fearful, and the simple fact that he is a child with little to no understanding of what is happening and why.

To compound the problem, that patient is often surrounded by pain, discomfort and fear from *several* different sources. In a given day, Audrey may have been awakened at 6:00 a.m. for a lab draw, requiring either a needle inserted into a vein or a finger poke. This was often followed by a trip to X-ray at 7:00 a.m. to be laid on a cold metal table, limbs strapped down, while they lowered a large camera to her tummy, often requiring me to leave the room. Many times, she had drainage tubes stitched to her skin, which pulled with each movement, not to mention open wounds, leaky ostomies or other secretions causing sores on her tender skin.

As mentioned before, she generally had some sort of dressing or bandage somewhere on her body that needed changed on a regular basis; this meant some sort of adhesive being removed from her skin almost daily. I think you get the picture! This kind of day is typical for so many patients, and it is vital to remember this and bring awareness of pain management to anyone involved with your child! If a nurse enters the room to start an IV in your child whose veins are difficult to access, it would be helpful for that nurse to know what other pain issues your child may have already experienced that day or even in the last 15 minutes! It may influence her approach to whatever care or procedure she must tend to for her already distraught patient.

Tips for Some Relief!

Learning tricks to minimizing pain and distress sometimes requires thinking outside the box. For example, one of Audrey's nurses placed a piece of central line dressing on herself to see which method of removal was the least painful. She learned that stretching the dressing out instead of up as it was removed eased the "pull" of the adhesive from the skin *(for tips on this simple step, see notes at end of book)*. We learned which ointments or warm moist cloth applications worked best for removing certain dressing types. We also discovered that if dressing packages were opened outside of Audrey's room, it lessened her distress about the procedure that was about to take place. This held true for any preparation required for an unpleasant procedure or care. Wound vac dressing changes were so stressful to her that we began preparing the supplies outside her room on a cart. We would then wheel the cart into the room, ready to proceed without delay, getting it over with as soon as possible!

The nursing staff will likely share with you signs to look for, which are indications of pain or discomfort, such as a high heart rate or high blood pressure readings on your child's monitor. These signs are especially important if your child is unable to express to you her pain level, whether she is an infant or an older child who is sedated. If your child is the age where she can use words to describe her pain, it might be helpful to involve Child Life to guide her in her description of pain. They may be able to introduce words that she can understand which may help her to communicate to you and the staff the way she is feeling, such as a "squeezing pain," using hand motions to enhance the description.

We learned that there are certain types of pains that are expected with a certain diagnosis, or following a particular procedure. Sometimes the pain our daughter was describing didn't seem to match the expectation. This called for us to probe further, until we could decipher the source of the pain that she was actually experiencing. It is important to not disregard a child's input about her pain, even if it might not make sense to the medical team.

Take note of the tolerance your child has in certain circumstances, whether it be for pain or discomfort, agitation or fear, etc. This will be different for every patient; if the staff caring for your child knows him as an individual versus just another patient, it will allow them to know how to meet his specific needs. You as the parent are the most important source for acquainting them with your unique child.

An example is Audrey's tolerance for lab draws versus IV insertions or shots. Lab draws *were* and *continue* to be such a regular part of her routine ever since she can remember, and she has developed coping skills to tolerate this discomfort with very little anxiety. Shots were another story when she was younger. While the pain was perhaps a little worse, but not by much, it required three of us - two nurses and me - to hold her down to administer shots!

Another procedure for which Audrey had very low tolerance was dressing removals. However, if she could be involved in the process, she did much better. So we put her in charge of removing or helping with removal of certain dressings.   She would apply the particular adhesive remover or cream if the dressing called for it. And then she would start pulling up a corner, and removing the adhesive in the manner that was least painful and the most manageable for her.

Knowing Audrey's low pain tolerance for adhesive removal, one of her nurses took the time to give her a bath and play dolls with her while the water soaked and loosened the tape around her IV so she could remove the dressing with the least amount of pain to Audrey. If that isn't a true depiction of compassionate nursing, then I don't know what is!

We realized that the most important way to help our child with her pain began with her care providers - *not only the medical staff, but us as well* - never becoming callous or accustomed to her pain; that there always be empathy and comfort lavished on her during her pain. Secondly, distraction and a relaxed atmosphere always helped to minimize the affects of pain and anxiety. Caregiving that involves gentleness and patience, being at ease, involving minimal people, diligence, and quick response will make a world of difference for your child's experience. And as mentioned before, the less pain and anxiety the patient endures, the more effective the healing process will be!

Knowing Medications and Their Effects -

Being well informed of pain medications, along with anti-anxiety drugs and sedatives will also empower you, as you strive to help manage your child's fears and pain. As you come to understand how your child reacts to certain medications, you will be able to share this insight with the different departments and staff members involved in your child's care, from the OR *(operating room)* to her hospital room.

Making personal notes and requesting the nursing staff to include in *their* reports reactions to certain drugs, effectiveness and dosing is a good start. This proactive approach could reduce unpleasant side effects and any unnecessary guesswork that might prove even dangerous to your child. As mentioned before, I am referring specifically to drugs such as sedatives, pain medications, anti-anxiety drugs given before or after a procedure - drugs whose doses are based on need or tolerance.

Benefits of Good Records –

Start keeping a record of the medications that have been administered to your child, the purpose of the medication, and how it affected your child. We came to learn that a certain anti-anxiety medication typically given pre-surgery would turn Audrey into a monster as the anesthesia wore off after surgery. Another sedative was so strong that she was "high" for hours! We were getting concerned, because she wasn't snapping out of it; she was just lying in her bed with a dazed look. Although it was effective in relaxing her, it was *too* effective, and we never used it again.

Be sure to include in your records additional medications administered in another facility, such as monthly IV infusions. It will be helpful to keep this record with you at all times in your billfold/wallet or whatever you carry with you. Anytime you enter a clinic or doctor's office, including dentists and eye doctors, the office will want to document all medications your child is taking and the accurate dosage in "mil equivalents". These measurements let the doctors know the concentration of each medication. I found it helpful to create a med chart on the computer, which made for easy updating. The other advantage to keeping this record with you is that in a time of distress when you are not thinking clearly, you don't need to worry about omitting any of this important information when giving your child's medical history. You may have committed to memory the dosages of each medication, but probably not the mil equivalents.

I also recommend keeping a record of any drugs administered in the past that are not current medications, including those given while in the hospital: sedatives, pain medications, anesthesia, etc. Be sure to note the dates administered, the purpose, and any side effects. This could be helpful information in the future.

In addition, always maintain a current record of vaccinations and immunizations your child has received. If there is one consistent record, there will be less discrepancy, especially if your child has received these inoculations from various clinics or doctors.

Along with this important data, it would be a good idea to maintain a record of surgeries and other procedures ever performed on your child, along with dates, the doctors' names and facilities. This information will likely be requested or needed in the future at some point! The best way to accomplish this is to request a copy of your child's medical records upon your departure from each hospital or clinic. These records may be lengthy, but you can refer to them for accurate dates and names as you create your own brief overview of her care. If you store this in your home file or folder along with her medication and vaccination records, you will have quick and easy access to it if you do ever need it.

Record types of supplies, i.e. dressings, creams, etc. *(including preferred brands!)* that have worked best for you and for what condition/situation. Note any items that did not work or that had adverse effects for your child, i.e. an allergic reaction. List the steps that were effective for certain procedures, such as a particular dressing change, the application of an apparatus like an ostomy bag - include the specific products with the steps. Not only will these notes be a helpful reference to you potentially in the future, but they may come in handy for someone else with the same needs! We often swapped ideas with other parents - those of us on the front lines sometimes have the best tips to share with each other! In fact, I was able to share some helpful problem-solving tips with a friend of my mother's who was having trouble with her ostomy.

Your accurate records and memory will serve as an important tool amongst any staff members and hospitals or clinics that are involved in caring for your child at any time. Again, having this documentation will ease your anxiety during a potentially critical emergency room visit or hospital admission, when all of this information is being requested of you - you can refer to your notes, or simply hand over your notes for them to make a copy!

You will likely be sent home with a folder containing pertinent information for follow-ups and home care. This might be a good place to store records of meds and procedures, etc. In my folder, I also taped business cards and recorded contact information of all the doctors, specialists, any hospital administration personnel involved in our case, etc. This was the best way for me to keep track of the names and phone numbers of staff members that I contacted on a regular basis. And, of course, I programmed the more frequent or urgent contacts in my phone so I always had them with me, i.e. her surgeons, doctors, hospital contacts, etc.

As a side note, it is also a good idea to keep with your med chart *(which is in your billfold!)* a note explaining your child's condition, along with doctor contact information in the event of an emergency. Include another personal emergency contact, as well, a spouse or other family member or friend. Most cell phones now have a feature that allows you to enter emergency information directly into your phone. Check with your phone service if you need help accessing this feature. I have recently done this on my phone, and I believe that emergency personnel are trained to check cell phones immediately for pertinent information.

It doesn't hurt to have emergency contact information in more than one place, though, in case your phone cannot be located – your billfold, your glove compartment in your vehicle, a laminated note attached to your child's car seat, etc.

JSYK

"Just so you know..."

Make personal notes for a filing or record system that might work best for you. (Note: I recommend starting a folder of information sooner than later, so that you have a place to file papers before you lose track of them.)

____
____
____
____
____
____
____

Start creating a list of medications your child has been given, including any notable side effects; you can use these lines here to begin, or a notebook you have already started for journaling.

____
____
____
____
____

_____

_____

_____

_____

_____

_____

_____

_____

_____

_____

_____

_____

_____

_____

_____

_____

_____

_____

_____

_____

_____

_____

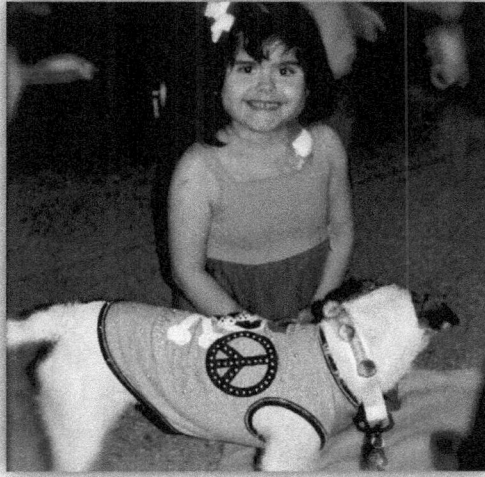

Chapter 7

Helping Your Child Cope

"Audrey endured enough hardship. We wanted to find ways to avoid any unnecessary pain and angst."

$\mathscr{F}$iguring out the best strategy to steer Audrey through this clinical experience was trial and error. The Child Life team gladly enlisted themselves to help us with the challenge, offering some creative and effective ideas. For example, we began having certain procedures done in her room instead of the treatment room. She was more comfortable in familiar surroundings; and it was such an ordeal to prepare to enter the treatment room and *then* get set up that she was inconsolable by the time the procedure got started! As mentioned before, we started prep-work *outside* her room, relieving her of a great deal of anxiety and anticipation of the impending procedure!

Boundaries for Your Child–
(And Gauging How to Handle Difficult Situations)

When coaching your child through difficult circumstances, it is best to consider your child's age, maturity level, and personality; also his state of physical, emotional, and mental health. If you are unsure how to handle a situation with your child, ask some of your nurses or the Child Life staff. They've been through this enough that they could offer some great advice! We also found it important to continue to set boundaries and to discipline when necessary. This can be tricky, because it is a delicate balance knowing the difference between willful behavior and drug-induced behavior. We also came to realize that, for Audrey, sometimes it was just "fed up" behavior from everything being done to her.

Our pediatrician offered some really helpful tips for handling belligerent behavior. One thing he suggested was stepping *away* and *out* of her room, to allow some time for her to cool off. So we would tell her that we were going to step out of the room until she calmed down; then we had to follow through immediately, without negotiating. Sometimes the situation required a nurse to go in the room instead of us; Audrey would occasionally respond better to someone other than her parents. And the nurse wasn't as emotionally involved, so she could offer a calming element to the tension; plus she was able to suggest a solution through new eyes.

If your child tends to physically lash out at the staff, it would be a good idea during your child's more reasonable moments to have an understanding but firm chat with her about how to treat her nurses. Several of Audrey's nurses commented on how often they were struck and kicked by a patient, while the parent failed to intervene. This behavior is unacceptable. There are other ways, much healthier means by which to channel a child's anger; but she needs the guidance of an adult to know how to manage this. Until she is taught, she won't know any better; she is just reacting in the moment.

A Time For Talk and A Time For Silence -

Audrey came to a point early on where she wanted to be informed of the details of her care - I think it helped her to prepare herself for anything potentially frightening or unpleasant. I can understand this because I am a planner, and I don't respond very well when things are suddenly sprung upon me - I need time to prepare.

She didn't like secrecy, and her intuition was ever accurate! She knew when something was amiss, so it was better to just be upfront with her. We also practiced discretion. We came to know what information she could and couldn't handle, when to share that information, how to share it, and how much to divulge. We would then guide the staff on how to do the same!

During the time that Audrey was sedated after her transplant, we were told by several staff members to read and talk to Audrey. I didn't realize before that when a patient is sedated, they drift in and out of consciousness, though it may not look as such. For this reason, I also suggest that whatever conversation is going on in your child's room, that the verbal exchange remain positive and hopeful as much as possible, whether she is conscious or sedated, two years old or twelve years old.

JSYK

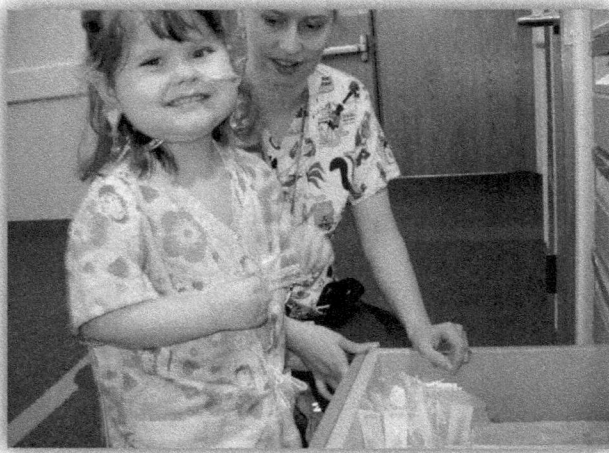

Audrey, dressed in scrubs that her nurse's mother made for her, helps Lisa gather supplies that are needed for a procedure.

Opportunities For Your Child to "Call the Shots!"

We also came to realize how important it was to give Audrey some control in her circumstances. This was another way of helping her to maintain her dignity as she became older. Often and for long periods of time she was bedridden and so dependent on others for almost anything. It was during her most intensive care that there seemed to be even more frequent and unpleasant encounters with staff, procedures, equipment, etc. So we became proactive in relinquishing some control to *her*, with positive results.

I created a large chart, with poster board and felt. I made cards with pictures of activities involved in her day, from bath time, to cares and vitals, doctor visits, play time, nap and story time, meal time...On the back I attached a piece of velcro, and on the chart I attached the matching piece with which to secure it. Each day, she could place the cards on her chart that she wanted for the day, creating, in a way, her own schedule. She could determine when she wanted certain cares or procedures to be completed, within a reasonable time frame. For example, perhaps she would choose her bath and vitals to be done after breakfast. She might place the playroom card right after her naptime. Audrey was three years old then.

An activity like this might serve well for younger ages, say between two and ten years of age. The Child Life personnel in your child's unit might offer some additional ideas for you, as well as other approaches for different ages.

Audrey understood there were certain cares that had to be completed, whether she liked them or not; but it helped her to be able to participate in those tasks. This might have included handing supplies to the nurses or to us during a dressing change, holding the thermometer when vitals were taken, assisting the nurse in gathering items from the supply cart or drawer, keeping her NG *(nasal gastric)* tube in place while we secured it to her face, etc.

We continued this routine at home - her involvement in her care. She would help wash her medicine syringes; I would place them in a tub of soapy water and she would swish them around - they were her "fishies"! It helped me and gave her something useful to do in a playful manner. She wanted to empty her own ostomy bag from time to time *(under supervision of course)*! She would hand us supplies during dressing changes, and help with hooking up her feeds or TPN. I think especially with older children or adults who are dependent on care, helping themselves is a valuable element to maintaining their dignity.

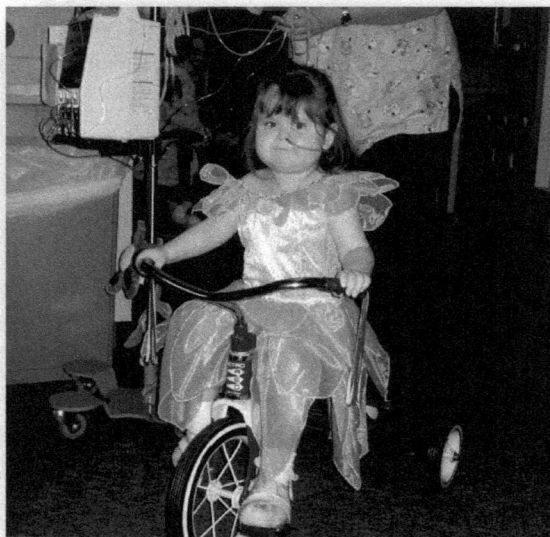

Audrey's first ride on a tricycle ...

Engage Your Child in Productive Activities-

I have mentioned activities we enjoyed and the creativity we employed. Make the most of not only *your* time but your child's time as well; by this I mean what they do with their time *and* with their mind will help them to better cope and to make the best of a situation from which they can't flee. Having something to concentrate on other than our troubles is a good distraction for the mind and soul - for *anyone*!

Some of the activities I listed in Chapter 2 as a way to "redefine normal" may serve as helpful ideas. I have also included other ideas

in *"Additional Tips"* at the end of the book. One of these is a game I created to give Audrey some mental therapy as well as occupational therapy; we "fished" for smiles! Instructions on how to make and play the game are found in that section.

There were times when Audrey was beside herself, especially in the PICU. By nature our daughter is one of the most easygoing and friendly people you will ever meet; loves interacting with others; finds a smile or laugh for just about any situation. But after days and weeks of overwhelming pain, prods, procedures, and people after groups of people in and out of her room for countless reasons at any hour, she had reached a point of not being able to cope anymore. That was when we had to step up and create a new twist in the care plan. Be aware, however, that a clever idea may not always be the ticket. There will be some days when nothing you try will help the situation. That's life for all of us, though. Don't let those days get you so down that you quit problem solving. As you continue to think of ways to help your child, that mental activity will help you, too!

Audrey also came up with other creative coping skills of her own. She was NPO *(no food by mouth)* for extended periods of time, both at home and in the hospital. The first few days were always the most difficult until her TPN *(central line nutrition)* kicked in. Even though she no longer had an appetite because of her IV nutrition, she still missed eating and tasting good food. So she began playing with food. Her favorite station in the playroom was the kitchen; she would enjoy "cooking" and serving a meal, we would have tea parties with "treats", she would even pack a "picnic" to have with her dad and I while we ate a real meal! *(We often received strange looks from other people...)*

She would play doctor and nurse with her babies and stuffed animals. They would have NG tubes, feeding tubes, ostomy bags and central lines that she had placed, and they would also get their vitals taken.

Even a few years after transplant and other medical procedures, she still plays hospital with her cousins and friends, really anyone she can recruit! When Audrey was three, we celebrated yet another birthday of *mine* in the hospital. She was NPO at the time, not allowed to eat, and on TPN for her sole nutrition. Her nurse shared with me something Audrey had asked her: "Mandee, may I have a popsicle? Tomorrow's my mom's birthday, and I want to give her a popsicle." It made me cry! My little girl couldn't enjoy a popsicle of her own in the heat of summer, so she wanted to give me what she considered to be the perfect gift!

Help Your Child Through Your Example!

Much of your child's experience as a patient will greatly depend on how you handle your circumstances and how you help him to handle *his* circumstances. Your demeanor and attitude, your confidence in his care, your anxiety level will all tend to reflect on your child's mood and how he reacts to situations and to the staff. If you are at ease, he will likely be more at ease, and this will really help him in many ways. He needs as much support emotionally and mentally as you do.

Let the Staff Get to Know Your Child and Family -

Another element of control is educating the staff on the most effective way to interact with your child. I commented earlier about cuing the nurses on the best approach to caring for Audrey. You know your child's personality and what she reacts favorably to and what upsets her.

Make a personality poster to put on your child's door, introducing the staff to their young patient. Consider writing from your child's point of view. If she is old enough she could give you input, or write it herself!

Include pictures of her doing normal activities at home. In fact, hang pictures all over the room! A respiratory therapist once told me that studies have shown when there are pictures of patients on display in their rooms, they receive better care from the staff. A patient, especially if sedated or really sick, may just be a body in a bed to a staff member. But that body takes on a personality when people see pictures of her active and interacting with loved ones. Her care then takes on an emotional aspect. This is yet another step in maintaining the dignity and value of that patient.

Your child could have fun creating a collage of pictures of herself, adding pictures from magazines depicting her favorite things. You could carry this one step further by letting your child find out about the people who take care of her. She could take *their* pictures and make another collage of the staff, depicting things that *they* like! They might discover some interests they have in common!

Instruct the staff on ways they may inform your child of a procedure that needs done, or the kinds of incentives or comforts that best fit his needs and personality. Offer ideas on how to relate with your child - mention his favorite cartoon characters, activities and toys. Maybe he gets upset when a team of half a dozen people suddenly descend upon him all at once. That can be intimidating for *any* patient, especially a *young* patient who is already scared and overwhelmed, and most likely mad at the world!

Request less people in the room - it's okay! We did, and the staff understood. Your team will likely work with you to put your child at ease and give him the best and most gentle care possible.

JSYK

"Just so you know..."

Try and see your child's experience through *his* eyes. Consider his fear, his discomfort and pain, his sense of feeling "caged"... Seek the nurses and their assistants for advice. For example, they helped me to understand the needs of a newborn - how to touch her, how to hold her, the signs of pain or distress, etc. Being knowledgeable of these tips helped me to better help my baby, and to be able to inform the nurse if I noticed something that needed attention.

What struggles is your child having regarding his hospital stay and condition? Have you sought out the expertise of the nurses, your pediatrician, or the Child Life staff?

_____

_____

_____

_____

_____

_____

_____

_____

What challenges are you having in handling a particular situation with your child? In what ways could you use some help or advice?

_____

_____

_____

_____

_____

Take some time to brainstorm some ways that might help your child to deal with his difficulties - or think of some questions to ask some staff members who may be able to offer solutions for you and your child.

_____

_____

_____

_____

_____

_____

_____

_____

_____

_____

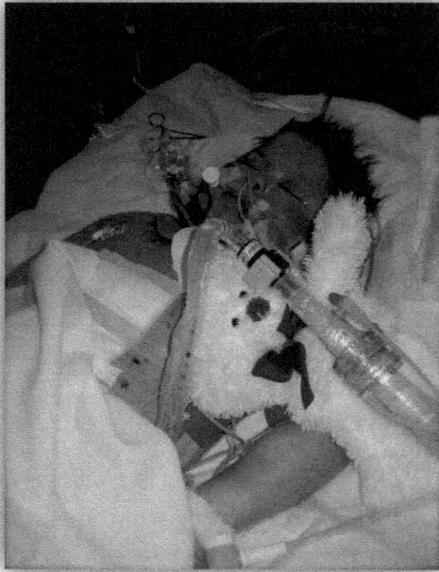

Audrey battled with Graft Vs. Host Disease
just two weeks after her transplant.

Preserving the Patient's Dignity-

Whether a patient is nine days old or nine decades old, they shouldn't lose their humanity once they are put in a hospital bed. When Audrey developed Graft vs. Host Disease after her transplant, an awful red blistering rash began to spread over every inch of her body, as I mentioned in Chapter One. This condition occurs in about five percent of organ transplant patients, and there is not a lot of knowledge about the disease at this point. At the onset of the rash, Audrey's skin would simply peel off with the removal of *any* adhesive, leaving open sores.

We couldn't even fasten her diaper. She had been sedated and intubated *(one of those "medical" words!)*. This meant she was on a ventilator, because her lungs had begun to fill with fluid, and shortly thereafter became the site for a fungal infection that was difficult to treat. Medications had caused excess fluid buildup in her body, leaving her swollen and "puffy." Her kidneys were shutting down, so she was put on dialysis.

Our hairdresser came and cut her hair to an inch in length, so we could apply a salve to the rash, which had spread all the way to her scalp. Her hair was greasy and spiked. It was a pitiful sight, to say the least!

But Audrey had a nurse with a nurturing spirit, who would wash her hair every morning and put a little bow in it. She would give her a bath, and change her linens. She would surround our little girl with her stuffed animals and decorative pillows, using them to prop up tubes and lines. And Audrey's pretty blankets would be neatly arranged on her bed. When we would enter her room in the morning, despite the red rash enveloping her entirely swollen body and her spiked hair soaked with greasy ointment, she would look like a little princess lying there!

On the other hand, there were days when we arrived, and noticed that nothing had been done for her to clean her up or to provide her with fresh linens *(this was when we were not allowed to stay in her PICU room)*. It seemed to say to us, "She's not even awake, in fact, she is barely there. She doesn't know any different, so why bother?" Her bed would be soaked and stained from her wounds, her ostomy bag, and other leaks or spills.

Obviously, these were the days that her nurturing nurse was not there. If both Dallas and I were there, or my mom or a friend, we could generally bathe her and change her bedding ourselves. The point is that her "nurturer" saw and treated Audrey as a sick little girl, not just a mass of tissue lying in a bed. She extended to Audrey some dignity in a very significant way.

When my grandmother was dying of pancreatic cancer, and she could no longer wash or dress herself, my mom and her sisters would bathe and dress her, and they would even fix her hair, and probably applied a little makeup to her face right up until her passing. Her body was perishing, but her inner person hadn't changed - she was still my grandmother, my mom's mother, a friend to many - not just a body. She had value as a human being, and deserved to be treated in such a way. Would her dignity have been as valued if she had been in an institution? My hope is that it would have been.

In her final weeks, my mother-in-law loved having fresh flowers in her room, and she craved watermelon - nothing else; so we made sure that she had fresh flowers and her watermelon.

My mom shares about her experience of having a certain personal procedure done. Without her permission or prior knowledge, the room filled with medical students, observing her in all her glory. Imagine how humiliating that would be - it was for *her* anyway!

As Audrey got older and more mature, reaching a higher level of understanding and discernment, the medical personnel who interacted with her took this into consideration, practicing good discretion when they entered the room or examined her. They were accommodating to us when we requested a limited number of staff members in the room at a time.

So, I encourage you as parents to help preserve your child's dignity while she remains in a position that leaves her very vulnerable. Invite the staff to join you in this endeavor by freely sharing any tips or insight that you think would prove helpful for them. They, in turn, will probably have some great suggestions themselves! Take advantage of their experiences and expertise!

JSYK

"Just so you know..."

It's heart wrenching to watch your loved one suffer. This reality seems magnified if she is looking neglected. Have you ever walked the halls of a nursing home and observed seeming neglect of some of the residents? ... Greasy hair, food-stained shirt, body odor, soiled rooms. Don't you just want to "fix it" for them? We can't make *everything* right for a person who is sick and suffering, but we sure can make *some* things right for them! Give your little princess a break from hospital attire if you can, and fashion a pretty dress around those tubes and wires. Brush her hair and put her favorite hairpiece in it, and paint her nails. Maybe your little guy wants to feel like a strong hero ... let him wear his Superman costume ... *and make sure he gets his baths!*

Note concerns and potential solutions that you have regarding your child's living situation - cleanliness issues, noise issues, lack of compassion or indelicate handling on the part of a staff member ...

_____

_____

_____

_____

_____

Brigitte D. Crist

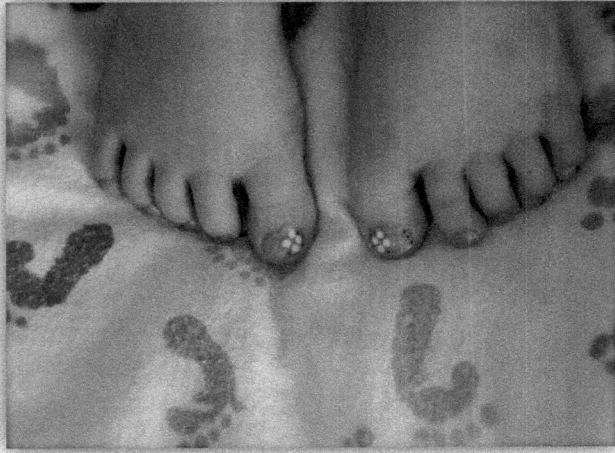

Chapter 8

"Take Care of Yourself"

"Come on my friend, let's take the stairs!"

𝒜 friend of mine at the Med Center snatched me away from the elevators one morning, as she spotted me about to board. This was *her* beck and call to me! So we climbed the stairs that morning, and, thanks to her, it became a daily habit for me.

About nine months after Audrey's transplant, I went for a complete physical for the first time in several years. I had lab work done, which revealed high cholesterol. My doctor suggested I take action, so I started watching my diet, but I didn't exercise as I should have.

Though it was difficult to fit an exercise routine into my schedule, and my energy level was very low, I should have made it a priority. However, a year later I had labs repeated, and my cholesterol level had dropped back down to normal.

I had *finally* gotten some exercise (by starting a gardening business!), I was eating a good diet, *and* I had lost ten pounds! I surmised that during the five years of extended hospital stays, my weight and my cholesterol level climbed to where they had never been because of the hours spent day after day sitting in a hospital room, and the number of meals I ate in the hospital cafeteria.

I could have done more exercising while at the hospital - taken the stairs more often, done some sit-ups in bed before turning in or getting up, not eaten nachos for a late night snack! Later on, I will offer some other lifestyle tips that I hope will help *you* to stay healthier.

Balanced Health–

Good health is not only physical. I am sure that you already understand this. I think, however, that when we are in a survival mode, we do just that - survive, not *live*. We eat in the cheapest or most convenient manner. We are also tired from physical and emotional strains, so we don't exert ourselves. We are also focused on the most urgent matter in our lives - a sickness, a trauma, a needy loved one - and we neglect our own needs and desires. This means our physical, emotional, spiritual, relational needs are often left unattended.

A great analogy is how the human body functions properly when all of its members are healthy. If all of the needs of a body are being met, and there is no damage, sickness, injury needing attended to, the body feels well, acts well, looks well, and all of the parts are being nourished as they should, able to contribute to a harmonious function of the body.

When Audrey was so sick with Graft vs. Host Disease, her vital organs needed extra help to continue functioning. Therefore all of the focus went to those organs. The team of doctors medicated her body so that the majority of the blood flow and oxygen were nourishing her sick vital organs. As a result, her limbs didn't receive the oxygen and blood flow they needed. They were being sacrificed to attend to the more vital members. Thankfully, she improved and there were no long term affects to the body parts that went without the life-giving blood and oxygen.

This is what can happen to us in a disaster. And if the conditions last too long, we suffer the consequences. It may be our health that suffers if we ignore it, it may be our relationships that suffer, because they are neglected. It may be our mental health that is affected, because we do not know how to deal with the tragic or taxing circumstances facing us.

Just as we had to seek professional help from the experts who know our child's condition, if we want to stay healthy or recuperate, we should seek out people who know how to help us in our specific trouble – maybe it's spiritual guidance and support, marriage and/or personal counseling, advice on staying fit and healthy physically, etc. My husband and I received some counseling as we prepared for Audrey's transplant. Looking back, we would have benefited from counseling from the very beginning of our ordeal. But of course we had no idea that it would still be going on several years later! If we would have known what we were up against, we would have sought out counseling long before we did - or forgone it all together and gone straight to a psychiatric ward!

JSYK

Nurture Yourself as You Nurture the Ones You Love!

In the middle of the crisis, we feel the need to be strong for our sick child or loved one and other family members. We consider it selfish to be fixing our eyes on ourselves and on our own needs. It took me awhile to figure this out. And when I did, it was very freeing. I began to understand that I shouldn't feel guilty for wanting to take care of myself. I finally realized that keeping myself healthy meant that I was more capable of tending to my daughter and her needs...

Just like those vital organs, which are responsible for keeping the body alive - when they were sick and not functioning properly the rest of the body suffered. You owe it to your loved ones to take excellent care of yourself so that you don't get sick, too; and so your relationships don't suffer undue neglect and strain during whatever crisis you are going through together. And remember, you are going through this *together*! Just like those body parts are working together and need each other, you need your loved ones to walk through your crisis with you. It's their crisis, too, so don't alienate them or isolate yourself.

I ended up in the emergency room once, and almost twice due to self-neglect and heavy stress. You want to be *proactive* rather than *reactive* to your health: Practice self-*maintenance* not self-*repair*, so you don't find yourself in the hospital as well!

You want to consider good health for the immediate benefit, which is keeping healthy and preserving your strength during the current crisis, but also think long-term; your loved ones will need you to be healthy for the long haul. I began to think about this: So, we get Audrey through her organ transplant, and then I come down with heart disease or cancer, and am unable to care for her properly.

Where does that leave Audrey and our family? Rest assured, self-care is not selfish, it is anything *but* selfish - you are doing it for your loved ones! They do *not* need another sick body to care for!!!

This realization made me think of the airline oxygen regimen in the event of a mid-air emergency. What is the rule of thumb for securing the oxygen masks? You, as a capable grown up, first apply *your* oxygen mask, then you will be empowered to help someone else put on his mask. If *you* collapse from lack of oxygen, you will be of no use to assist anyone else.

Practical Steps to Self Care -

Nutrition

Beverages -

When I landed in the emergency room, part of my ailment was dehydration. As a result, they had to hydrate me by way of IV. I highly recommended that you hydrate *yourself* - with H2O! You may think me over the top, but I kept a bottle of lemon or lime juice at the hospital to spritz my water. It adds a little flavor and is so refreshing! Indulge in a bottle of club soda along with an unsweetened power juice, such as cranberry or pomegranate. Just add a splash of juice to your club soda, and you have a healthy "grown-up" treat! If you consume soda after soda, consider what you are putting in your body. It's packed with sugar, chemicals, *and* sodium!

Keep a large water cup or bottle with you. Request a pitcher for yourself, and keep it filled. Hopefully your hospital offers water dispensers that are self-serve. If not, don't hesitate to ask for refills when you need them. The hospital staff understands the importance of hydration. It is my experience that the larger the cup I have within reach, the larger the quantity of water I will consume! I set a goal for myself: *"Make sure to empty that cup at least twice a day."*

Coffee:

Limit your intake, and limit the additives! If you generally use two packets of sugar, try reducing it to one, or if you now use one packet, try reducing it to half a packet. When I was able to, I kept a supply of my own milk or half and half instead of the powdered cream. It tastes better to me, and I figure the real thing is probably healthier.

When considering creamer, remember that the flavored ones have lots of sugar and preservatives! I also used whole milk, when available, vs. half and half - less calories! For flavor, sprinkle some cinnamon in your coffee -a healthy alternative and immune booster! You could go one step further, and keep a bottle of vanilla extract on hand for a touch of sweetness without the sugar.

Soda:

Make soda a treat, not a staple. For example, make a pact with yourself to only have soda on pizza and movie night, and maybe Fridays at lunch. You will feel better physically, and I guarantee you will feel better mentally - another element of control! You will know you've taken another big step in self-care! By now, you probably have gained a friend in one of your child's nurses and are starting to confide in her. Ask her to hold you accountable! Make it fun - maybe she'll suggest a penalty if you slip!

Diet -

If your child frequents the hospital or is inpatient for extended periods, it is important for *you* to eat right. After Audrey's birth and subsequent complications, I treated myself to a donut every morning for breakfast in the hospital cafeteria. And then I returned to my daughter's bedside and sat most of the day. I was still wearing maternity pants six months after giving birth! I think my attraction to the donut was "comfort food". I have read that when under stress, sugars and carbohydrates are craved by our bodies. I think that if our bodies are accustomed to these foods, they are probably craved even more. If you condition your body to consume healthier items, you will acquire more of a taste for good foods, and your body won't crave the sugars and fats as much. I have learned this by experience!

When we returned for other hospital stays, I brought in a lot of our own food. I kept nonperishable foods on hand in a picnic basket in the room. Even as a decoration, the picnic basket made our small abode look more homey! Thankfully, our room had a refrigerator, too. I'd like to share some menu ideas that are practical and feasible in the hospital.

Menu Ideas -
Simple ... Quick ... Cheap ... Healthy ... Tasty

Mixed greens with a protein on top:
Purchase pre-cooked chicken or shrimp, or top with tofu or cheese - cubed or shredded. Keep a box of croutons, some mini carrots, cucumber slices, and naturally low-fat dressing: Choose one with olive oil or other healthy oil - my favorite is a balsamic vinaigrette, because the balsamic vinegar is so savory, in and of itself.

Then you won't need to load on the salt or other unhealthy flavor enhancers! Add a whole grain baguette on the side, and your vinaigrette can double as a dipping sauce!

The great thing about a meal like this is that besides being nutritional, it is quick and easy. You can keep all of the ingredients in the fridge, ready to go - enough to last three or four meals; all of the ingredients will stay fresh for a few days. A salad makes a quick lunch *or* dinner.

Whole grain breads with sandwich fixings:

Choose sandwich bread, hoagie or hamburger buns, flat buns, wraps - or a variety! Keep a weekly supply of deli meats on hand. If you buy the prepackaged deli meat, you may be getting more preservatives, but *wait!* - You *also* get a handy storage container with the deal - and those *do* come in handy! Italian meats will keep longer, and they make for a fun and flavorful sandwich or wrap. Dress it with the vinaigrette used for your salad, and then use some of your salad as a topping - I love the crunch of cucumbers on my sandwiches! Provolone cheese is great on Italian sandwiches and mozzarella is fairly low in sodium.

BBQ Sandwiches:

On the buns or hoagies you purchased for your other sandwiches, switch the menu around for one meal and have barbeque! In most deli sections, they offer prepackaged and precooked barbeque meats - all you have to do is heat it up. They generally have a selection of beef, pork, and chicken. Add a container of coleslaw or your favorite potato salad, some baked potato chips, fruit, and *that* is a meal worth skipping the cafeteria for!

Add some life to your existence and pack your picnic basket with your tasty BBQ, and find a scenic picnic spot - it could be in the lobby by a fake waterfall and indoor tropical plants!

Include a tablecloth with your staples, and make the ambience a little more pleasing! I would even tote along the fresh flowers I brought from my garden - your husband *may* roll his eyes, but just imagine that he secretly enjoys the fuss as well ... perhaps he really does!

Pre-Cooked Pastas:
These can be found in the deli department, i.e. tortellini or ravioli. This is not the least expensive menu choice, but a nice treat.

Topping ideas:
- *Jar of marinara sauce or pesto*
- *Mozzarella cheese – fresh, block, or shredded*
- *Favorite fresh herbs sprinkled on top (for a touch of elegance that is pleasing to the eye and to the soul - a welcome change from a sterile hospital setting!)*

Cheese & Veggie Tray: Can be used as a side to your pasta dish or by itself for snacks or a light meal.
- *Cucumbers, grape tomatoes, and other veggies*
- *Olives*
- *Chunks or slices of cheeses*
- *Favorite crackers (again, check sodium level; include whole grain)*

Store either in a divided container or individual containers. These items can also be tossed on your pasta, your sandwiches, or salads. They are a good staple to have on hand.

Trail Mix:

Mix your favorite nuts and dried fruit together and fill snack bags for an easy and portable munchie. If you must have some chocolate, mix in a few semi-sweet or dark chocolate morsels - which will contain less sugar than candy-coated chocolate pieces.

Add some cereal, small carton of milk, and fruit to your shopping list, and you have groceries for about a week - *if* you're willing to eat leftovers! Whole grain bagels and veggie cream cheese double as breakfast *and* lunch; you could even slap on a slice of your deli meat to carry you further to the next meal.

When we were in the hospital so much, these few meal ideas offered several benefits: a touch of *partially* homemade cuisine, nutritious ingredients, little prep time, a tasty and inexpensive alternative to eating out or cafeteria food, and leftovers that were easy to store for another meal.

A Word of Caution: When choosing prepackaged items, remember that the sodium content will likely be higher. Keep this in mind as you are watching your health. You don't want your blood pressure to escalate in the process! Remember that the menu in the cafeteria is also probably packed with sodium. Just be cautious and practice moderation.

As far as cafeteria meals, the more frequent ones I ate were breakfasts, and this is why:

- My daughter had company while the nurses were doing her morning cares.
- It is generally the least expensive meal to eat in the cafeteria.

- At the Med Center, they offered some killer omelets - large enough to save the other half for the next day!
- Breakfast foods are generally hearty and filling - a good way to start the day, and better to eat this way in the morning, so you can work it off by *climbing the stairs all day!*

Just some ideas ... take 'em or leave 'em!

JSYK

Exercise!

I am serious about climbing the stairs! It's a great cardiovascular workout along with muscle toning. Take frequent breaks when you can to stretch, get your heart pumping, your blood flowing, and clear your head.

Emotional, Mental, and Spiritual Well-being -

Isn't it said, "When life gives you lemons, make lemonade"? Another version is, "When your child is sedated in the PICU, catch up on your sleep!" Because you will need it later! Curl up in a chair and enjoy a good book or magazine - it will keep your mind from wandering to where it shouldn't. Take a jaunt to the gift shop and find a notebook to start journaling! While you're there, pick up a puzzle book. My husband and I found math puzzles to be an enjoyable and productive way to pass the time - we were doing something together, and solving other problems outside of *ours.* Such an activity is a healthy exercise for one's mental state as well as one's soul!

You need more than good nutrition and rest. You have emotional needs, psychological needs, mental needs, spiritual needs. Don't neglect them.

"Guilty Pleasures"

Shortly after Audrey's "Big Surgery" *(the last major surgery before her transplant)*, when she was not doing well, *I* was not doing well either, and my big need at the moment was a latte. I went through this dilemma of guilt: Do I leave my daughter's side to go help myself to a latte? Am I being inconsiderate to think of a treat to myself while my daughter fights for her life? So I analyzed it ... *or* justified it: I would get some exercise, a chance to stretch and take some deep breaths, a comforting drink that would warm me up in the frigid hospital conditions, something tasty that would do my soul good. I could then return refreshed and ready to tend to my daughter once again. So I went and got the latte!

If you are not sure how to take care of *your* needs or where to start, I suggest that you make a list of things that are important to you, things which bring you peace and perhaps renew your energy. These may include a stroll in a garden or a visit to an art museum, some quiet time at the start of the day, a vigorous run, having tea with a friend, time to read, watching a ball game, scrapbooking, or doing something productive - I know this is especially important for men; I've witnessed it firsthand!

Here is a sample from my list, which may spawn some ideas for you:

Writing - I love to create in many different ways. One way is with words; it allows me to express and sort out my thoughts and feelings, to document moments I want to remember, and to problem solve, all the while doing something I love.

Beauty and Aesthetics - When my surroundings are enhanced with beauty and order, it brings me peace. I nest at home, I nest in our hospital room, I nest in my vehicle and in a hotel room! In the summer, I would decorate our room with an ongoing stock of fresh cut flowers from our garden. I used baskets to store some of our things, which added a touch of warmth to the room. I also politely created a separate place for the nurses' supplies and our medical supplies so they weren't scattered hither and yon.

I couldn't live in cluttered and junky looking surroundings. I also brought blankets and pillowcases from home for Audrey's bed as well as mine. We made our beds everyday, and neatly arranged our pillows and her stuffed animals. It was also a great way to maintain routine, and to continue her responsibilities of picking up after herself, as she would do if she were at home.

Art - I also enjoy photography, painting and sketching, writing music and prose, and designing. This is all a great outlet for me, something that brings me satisfaction and joy. What I wouldn't have given to have a music room in the hospital where I could run and pound out my fears and frustrations on a grand piano!

In the evenings, after getting Audrey tucked in for the night, I would saunter out to the ... "er" ... *my* waiting room. There, I would do my thing well into the night. I also had a small reading lamp, so some nights I would just stay in her room and write on the computer. I did minimal web surfing, because I found I would spend *way* too much time very easily.

Walking - During my *"swingin' single"* stage of life, I used to walk everyday in a picturesque park filled with large trees along a winding sidewalk, all nestled amongst turn-of-the-century homes. In the hospital, Audrey and I would walk down one hallway to the elevator, then up the elevator to another hallway. We would, however, run into lots of friends to visit with on our escapades, and we always found our way to the gift shop, the fish tanks, and the river!

Coffee – I have mentioned this one a few times already, haven't I? Well, I wasn't a coffee drinker until I spent two years in Colombia, South America, where I discovered "cafe con leche." The closest replica I can find here in the States is an expensive latte! *(At home I can make it myself)*. My mother would usually give me a coffee shop gift card when we were in the hospital for more than a week or so. And that was my treat to myself. Someday I'd like to do the same for others who enjoy coffee like I do! Remember what I suggested earlier about your coffee indulgence - limit your calories! And only order that fancy coffee laced with sugary syrup once in a *great* while! Be a purist - stick to simple *fresh* coffee and milk!

JSYK

"Just so you know..."

Eating healthy will not only keep your body happy and feeling well, but it will also help you to stay healthier mentally and emotionally! And I don't need to tell you how that can help you in your circumstances. We need all the help we can get in *all* areas!

It may be difficult to consider taking care of yourself as a self*less* act rather than *selfish*.   But we are living beings who need maintenance to function well - your car needs fluids and fuel, good tires, a good "once over" every several months. Don't you take care of your vehicle for *your* benefit more than for the vehicle's sake? After some use, your cell phone needs charged, because *you* depend on it – just as *you* need charged to keep going for those who depend on *you*!

In what ways are you already taking care of yourself?
(Give yourself some credit!)

_____

_____

_____

_____

_____

_____

How can you improve your diet? How can you realistically fit in some exercise?

_____

_____

_____

_____

_____

_____

What feeds your soul?
(Gardening, yard work, tinkering in the garage or on a project, watching sports ...)

_____
_____
_____
_____
_____

_____
_____
_____
_____

When is a good time for you to fit these things into your day?

_____
_____
_____
_____
_____
_____

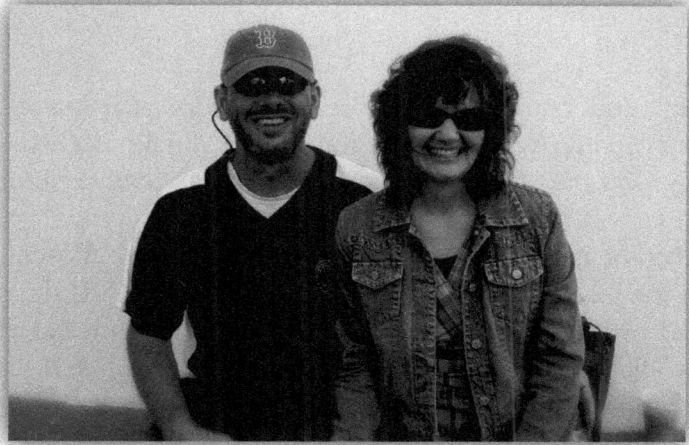

Chapter 9

Preserving Your Relationships

"A stroll through the park, dinner and a movie, a night at home ..."

*D*allas and I had been married a whopping four and a half months when our adventure began. We were still getting acquainted and adjusting to life together. Over the course of the next few years, I slowly learned that people cope with crises very differently, namely my husband and I. In talking with and observing other families, I found it was the case for them as well.

A Team of Two Distinct Individuals!

After seven or eight months of our *first* extended hospital stay, Dallas started staying home some evenings. To be honest, I felt like he was losing interest – in me, in Audrey, in our family.

I didn't understand why he would choose to stay home and not spend the evening with Audrey and me. It finally occurred to me *(probably a couple of years down the road during our next long-term stay)* that he was tired.

Neither of us was ever home, except to sleep. When Audrey returned for hospitalizations after release from the NICU, she had graduated to the Pediatric floor, so I could stay with her at night. Dallas would work a long, exhausting eight, nine or ten hour day, and then come straight to the hospital until it was about bedtime - night after night, week after week, month after month...He never complained about it, he just stayed home when he needed to. And he *needed* to from time to time! This whole ordeal took such a toll on us physically, emotionally, mentally, and relationally. We had to take time out and time away once in awhile - and so do you, sometimes alone and sometimes with the important people in your life.

Dallas more readily recognized when he needed a break, and took it without remorse. I, on the other hand, always felt guilty leaving Audrey at the hospital - even if I was leaving her with a friend or staff member. I felt selfish and irresponsible as a parent. So, sometimes I didn't leave, or I postponed a meal. And then I would get tired, hungry, and cranky, and that sure wasn't any help to Audrey *or* her nurses.

My husband was a rock through our trying times, I think partly because he knew when he'd had enough and when he needed to walk away for awhile. He also doesn't panic like I do, and so he reacts to situations a little more calmly. This is a strength he adds to our relationship - a strength that helped carry me much of the time.

The other thing that I learned about my husband was that during a stressful situation, he doesn't do well with other people around, including family members - the larger the crowd the higher his stress and anxiety level. It helped me to have friends and loved ones around, especially during a critical stage in Audrey's condition. They helped keep my mind occupied and my worry at bay. To some extent, they *lowered* my stress and anxiety level, and I valued their support. When my husband felt like being alone and quiet, they were there for me to talk to and to keep me company. Neither of us was right or wrong; it was just important to try and understand one another and strive to help meet each other's emotional needs. Sometimes that meant letting other people help or keeping them at a distance when necessary.

You may deal with your situation in an entirely different way than other members of your family. This is to be expected, because we are each unique individuals with distinct personalities and ways of coping. The benefit is that you can use your differences to help each other and to lend each other strength where you each are lacking, and to encourage one another.

On any given day, one of you may need to uphold the other because of a particularly difficult time. The next circumstance may perhaps present an opportunity for your partner or loved one to be the strong one for *you*. It is important that you share and respect each other's struggles and point of view.

If your partner requires time alone, then support him in that. After taking the time he needs, he will likely return with a fresh perspective and renewed energy to be of more help to you and your sick child.

The Nurturer vs. the Hunter ...

Understand that it may be difficult as a man to sit or wait for a very long period of time, feeling as though he is doing nothing. As a woman, nurturing may come naturally to you, and you know how to tend to your child's needs *while* you sit and wait. A man may be climbing the walls, not knowing what to do, how to contribute. He has put his "hunt and gather" instincts on hold, and feels of no use! So send him to "hunt" for some dinner or coffee. Let him "gather" the newspaper to occupy his mind and his time! Allow him to go home and mow the lawn - in this way he is able to work out any frustration with aggression on the ever-forgiving grass and mower, not the doctor with a poor bedside manner. It also makes him feel like he is doing something worthwhile!

Husbands, a word to the wise for you! Your lovely wife may have been endowed with the gift of nurturing and the patience of Job. While you so adore these qualities and appreciate the loyalty and nobility of motherhood, this is what will also get your goat when she won't leave your child's bedside to go on a date! You've had enough of the hospital and would like to enjoy a night out with your wife's undivided attention, and she doesn't seem to share the same sentiment. May I suggest that you let it go and take a rain check - go see that "shoot 'em up" flick by yourself that she wouldn't like anyway. In a day or two, offer to sit with your child while she has lunch with a friend. After she feels more comfortable being away for a short time, she will be ready for that date.

Wives, did you just read that? Appeal to your husband's need for time alone with you. If you aren't acquainted enough with your child's nurses or care partners to feel comfortable leaving your child strictly in their care, then ask a trusted family member or friend to come and sit with her while you and your husband get away together.

Let each other know that you are not forgotten, and share some much needed love and attention. Your marriage needs continued nurturing just as your sick child does! Don't put your relationship on the back burner; it needs to be especially strong during this difficult period. Family time with your other children is vital, too, but don't substitute those family times for date night.

Perhaps you've gotten acquainted with another family during your stay. Plan a double date some night - it would be a great opportunity to share experiences, swap helpful tips, or just have a nice evening out and some diversion from life in the hospital. My experience has been that this setting also fosters conversation that might not have happened with just the two of us.

Talk!

And speaking of conversation, it is important that this exercise also take place between just the two of you at least some of the time. If something is bothering you, speak up! It has taken me a long time to figure this out. I tend to keep things inside, not feeling the right to be "objectionable." I stew instead! Had Dallas known how important family support was to me in Audrey's critical times, maybe he would have been more tolerant of their company!

If you have a conflict, always try to reconcile. You may need to walk away and take some time to consider how to reconcile and what words to use, rather than spilling your frustrations, anger, and accusations in the heat of the moment. Write your partner a note - a kind note, a note saying: "I'm sorry" or "I appreciate and love you." Leave it on his/her pillow to find later that night. During Audrey's six-month stay in 2006, our lives were bombarded with trial after trial after trial. Our marriage really took some serious hits! Our anniversary that summer was spent yet again in the surgery waiting room. I still have the card Dallas gave me that year. His message inside reads, *"Hang in there with me and we'll pull through everything! Love you very much, Yours ..."*

JSYK

"Just so you know..."

Hard times test relationships. If you don't pull together you will pull apart. Taking time for each other will make it easier to stay close. Extending attention, affection, and support to one another will create a stronger buffer for the conflicts to penetrate when they arise!

It might help for you to jot down some thoughts concerning your relationship with your spouse or other loved ones. Perhaps note some struggles or misunderstandings, neglect or hurts that need to be reconciled. Equally important would be to make a note of some ways you could show love and appreciation to your support team - spouse or other family members/friends, considering the present challenges you are facing as a couple, or with your child's condition, or within your family structure.

_____

_____

_____

_____

_____

_____

_____

_____

_____

_____

_____

_____

_____

_____

_____

_____

_____

In what ways can your partner show you support? What do you need from him/her right now that would lift your spirits and provide some emotional strength for you? Can you share this with your partner? He or she may be searching for ways to help you, but just doesn't know what you need!

_____

_____

_____

_____

_____

_____

_____

Brigitte D. Crist

_____
_____
_____
_____
_____
_____
_____
_____
_____
_____
_____
_____
_____
_____
_____
_____
_____
_____
_____
_____

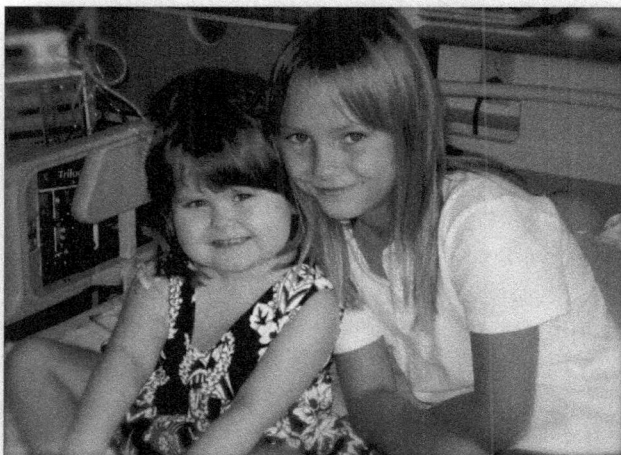

Chapter 10

Keeping your Family Intact

"Let your family know you are all in this together; it's their mission for the moment - choose to accept it and embrace the challenge!"

It might be the tendency of other children to feel neglected while their sibling is receiving so much attention from their parents and others during a hospital stay or a chronic condition at home. Just as with your hospitalized child, it would be beneficial to maintain the other children's routine as much as you can. This trial is a hardship on them as well. When you are able, continue with family activities. As I have already mentioned, there is a certain security in a "normal" routine and schedule, and it will reassure your other kids that they are still loved and are just as important to you as your child who is hospitalized.

In our case, Audrey's older sister, Teryn, lived several hundred miles away. With Audrey's frequent hospitalizations, we weren't able to see her as often as we would have liked. At Teryn's young age, it was probably difficult to understand this. It may have looked to her as our full attention and love being directed at Audrey. When she was able to visit, we tried to include her in our life at the hospital as much as possible. For her sake, we needed to spend time with her away from the hospital as well. The balancing act was never ideal for any of us, but we did our best and it worked out.

Involve them in their sibling's care. They can be of help at whatever maturity level or age they may be. It could be as simple as playing a game with their sibling, filling her glass with iced water, fetching a towel or needed supplies, painting her toenails or giving her a foot massage... The options for serving are endless. It can create a bond amongst all of the family members, forming a team atmosphere. Common goals are the result, causing the family to pull together. The focus is taken off an individual and placed on the family unit and desired end. Maybe that end is getting their sibling back home, or meeting a certain milestone in physical therapy, or getting rid of a line or a pump or a tube!

In my experience, children generally rise to the occasion when they feel needed or realize that they can be useful! Audrey's little cousins and friends would faithfully remember to pray for her everyday. Her cousin, Micah, was three when she began to pray for "Baby Audrey" each day; and she did this for probably two or three years!

Several of Audrey's little friends even paid her visits. Other little ones on our email update list learned at a very young age about praying for a sick friend, making her cards, sending thoughtful gifts...

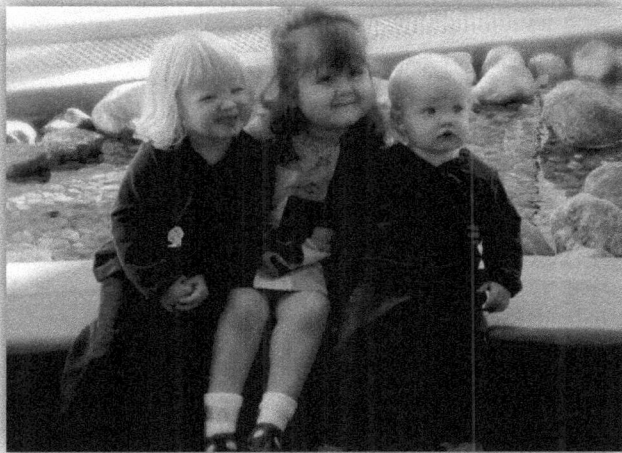

*Audrey, age three, hangs out with cousins,
Lanie and Ellie, by the "river."*

In turn, your child who is hospitalized can make his own contribution to the team. It might make him feel good to be able to explain to his brother or sister how a certain machine works, or what ingredients make up his IV or TPN fluids and how they nourish the body. It may be giving a family member or even friend a tour of the floor or hospital, introducing them to his nurses and other "buddies" on the staff.

He will have the unique opportunity to witness firsthand other children going through sicknesses and struggles of their own. He may even get the chance to reach out to some of these kids, while perhaps looking past his own challenges for a change!

Perhaps you can still have your family movie night in his room, with popcorn and the works! If you have young children who aren't allowed in the unit, see if you may borrow a room outside the unit for your family event. Order in pizza! Create a fun atmosphere for the entire family when possible. During Audrey's first Thanksgiving, the NICU staff allowed our family to use a room just off the unit for our holiday dinner, allowing Audrey to join us. It was a very thoughtful gesture on their part.

When your child's condition is perhaps more critical, think of other ways to still involve the family. Maybe the siblings or cousins can make cards and pictures to send in to her. If you think it appropriate, take photos or video in your child's hospital room and share them with family members in the waiting room. If you have access to a web camera, communicate with the family via computer from your child's room to home or wherever the family may be.

If a holiday is approaching, involve your family in making some decorations to put up in her hospital room. Create a mural of pictures - family and friends to hang on her wall. One year, I decorated Audrey's IV pole with strips of white and red paper to create a candy cane look for Christmas. With each season, we decorated her window with window clings or cutouts made from tissue and construction paper - autumn leaves, Christmas scenes, spring flowers and Easter eggs, etc. One of the moms I became acquainted with had a good old-fashioned Valentine-making party in her daughter's room.

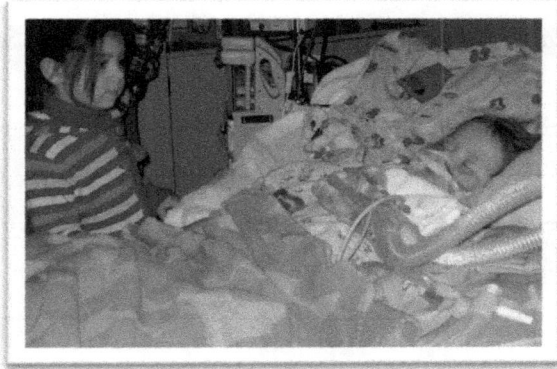

*Audrey's friend, Darcie, visited her on Valentine's Day.
At age five, she held Audrey's hand for the better part of half an hour,
and sang to her.*

JSYK

"Just so you know..."

Facing this challenge together as a family can provide a great opportunity for your kids to learn about selfless giving and responsibility, as well as differences in people. It may allow them to see disabilities or sicknesses in others with more empathy. It is also a chance to strengthen family ties by working together to make it through a hardship.

The experience can also provide some inspiration for them to help other sick kids later on! Perhaps one day, their school or a community group in which they are involved could deliver toys, movies, or activities to the pediatric floor for other children going through hard times.

How can you involve your family in your present circumstances?

_____

_____

_____

_____

_____

_____

_____

_____

What are family members struggling with? What are some ways to help meet their needs? How can you help your other children to feel secure by preserving some elements they are familiar with – routines, surroundings, other loved ones they are comfortable with?

_____

_____

_____

_____

_____

_____

_____

_____

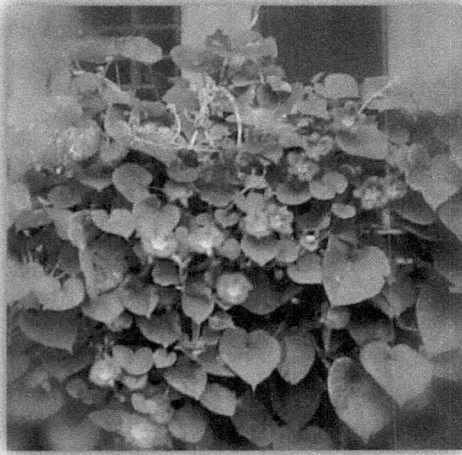

Chapter 11

Dealing with the Rollercoaster of Emotions

*"When emotions hit out of the blue, you are not losing it...
It really is to be expected!"*

*"I don't like living life in a glass house. When I'm having a hard
day and can't seem to keep it together, there is no place to escape the
public eye to just have a moment of privacy and break down. I'm
tired of the surgical team seeing me in my p.j.'s in the morning as I
groggily try to engage with them - I was up yet again until midnight
or so writing, and then up several times throughout the remainder of
the night to change a diaper, or silence a beeping pump, or chase a
student or surgery resident out of the room!"*

Journal Entry   November 2, 2006

(A few months later...)

> "Extreme anxiety and stress can drain you of energy,
> concentration, memory, patience, ambition and
> drive, and the overall ability to cope and function as
> you should. I try with all my might not to let it rob
> me of my joy."
>
> *January 1, 2007*

I thought it might help you to read some excerpts from my journal to take you back to a time when I was in your shoes. The first entry was written on our way to Colorado to attend the memorial service for my mother-in-law, Camilla. About the time that Audrey was hospitalized for a six-month stay in the spring of 2006, Camilla had been diagnosed with stage-four cancer. When she took a turn for the worse in September, Dallas went out to be with her for about three weeks. She passed away shortly after his return trip home. My mother came to stay with Audrey in the hospital, so that he and I could return to Colorado for the funeral.

Bad news may seem to be stalking you, while a storm of miserable circumstances hails on you. I think my husband and I both wondered at times when it would stop. Would we ever catch a break? We finally did . . . it was a few years down the road, but we *finally* did. There *is* a light at the end of the tunnel for you, as well.

JOYK

Symptoms of When You've Just Had Enough!

Memory and Concentration –

Have you had lapses in your memory in which you can't remember where you placed your car keys or where you parked in the hospital parking garage three days ago? Have you ever forgotten your ATM pin code during a crisis? What about your social security number or anniversary date?

These can be sure symptoms of overload - overload of stress, trauma, information, one dire situation after another... I know! In a period of about one week I experienced every single one of these! Audrey had maxed out her health insurance coverage *just* before another major surgery. We were informed of this *after* the surgery! We even inquired about coverage *before* the surgery, and were informed that, yes, there was still coverage on her policy. You can imagine my panic, as my life flashed before my eyes, homeless and on the street corner, begging for pennies to cover Audrey's medical costs!! Well, thankfully she qualified for Medicaid, which meant interviews and mountains of paperwork to be filed. On my interview, I couldn't remember my social security number that I've known since the 6th grade; I couldn't remember our wedding anniversary date, I got my husband's birthdate wrong and had to correct it. One day I went to the ATM, and instead of drawing out cash, I drew a total blank on my passcode!

Where's the Paper Bag?!?!

Perhaps you have even had anxiety attacks. I remember one instance in the hospital elevator. My heart started racing, a sense of claustrophobia came over me, and I began to sweat, feeling like I couldn't   breathe.   Maybe you feel tense all the time, like an overwound rubber band that could snap at any time or a pressure cooker about to blow its top! And maybe sometimes you *do* - snap or blow. It may be at your spouse or other loved one, or a staff member. After you have had time to process your fit of rage, you wonder why you reacted so strongly.

I think for me anxiety would build up, leading me to get easily annoyed or impatient when things didn't go right (or my *perception* of "right!"). That often led me to get angry in situations where I wouldn't *ordinarily* get angry. Those were moments when I would go for a walk, or find a piano if I could – stepping away from the circumstances for a short while helped to calm me down. If I were unable to step away at the time, I would pray as hard as I could, and take some deep breaths ...

Just Breathe!

Deep breathing is an effective technique used in yoga and other exercises and therapies. This practice offers the body all kinds of health benefits on many levels - physical, psychological, spiritual, emotional. Taking in deep breaths introduces large amounts of oxygen into the blood stream and lungs, which is vital to good health, flushing out toxic carbon dioxide. It can help the body to relax and get re-centered. My mother recently had foot surgery, and the nurses instructed her to take deep breaths as a way of relieving her anxiety before the anesthesiologist put the mask on her face. It has been said that too often our bodies don't receive enough oxygen to maintain good health. Try finding a quiet place - like the hospital chapel or garden - and take time to just breathe deeply, slowly, in through the nose and out through the mouth.

When the Honeymoon is over, and You've Become Territorial!

Have you bristled, because yet another staff member just wandered in the room, while you were having some family time together? This may not happen until a month or so down the road. But after some time, as you try to carry on with daily life in somewhat of a commune, it's bound to get to you. The nursing staff may leave supplies lying around, causing the room to look out of order and it really miffs you! There are potentially simple solutions to help you deal with these frustrations. Feel free to be honest with the staff, and like we had to do, schedule some private family time, when you do not want to be disturbed except in an emergency. Make it known to the staff, and post a sign on the door. You also may need to post a schedule for visitors if you are receiving guests at inopportune times. If you are sending news to friends and family members, updating them on your loved one's progress, this would also be a great venue for advising them of the visiting hours that you have arranged.

As far as *your* room versus *their* room … Try to understand that the nurses and other staff regard the patient rooms as their work area, and rightfully so. Unless they have ever had a loved one in the hospital or been a patient themselves, most of them don't even consider that your child's room has become home to you for the time being. They don't mean to disrespect your privacy or clutter and mess up *your* space.

It is possible to tactfully and kindly make your sentiments known. If you don't feel comfortable speaking directly to the nurses, share your feelings with someone you trust so that they may inform the nursing staff. This person could be a charge nurse, social worker or chaplain. Once the staff understands your perspective, they will likely be more considerate. You as the concerned caregiver can offer solutions.

Delegate one area of the room for supplies. I even brought plastic containers into the hospital for organizing supplies. Empty tissue boxes work, too! Solicit the techs or care partners to help the nurses in cleaning up after themselves and returning things to their rightful place. Your child as the patient might even want to help. This would be another way to involve him in his own care, assigning him an "important" task! And children generally enjoy teaming up with their nurses and care partners. They were Audrey's best friends! She always looked forward to doing something with them, and it strengthened the bond and trust she had with them.

JSYK

The Conflict With Gratitude and Guilt...

I found myself struggling with this inner turmoil of mixed emotions. On a given day, we could be receiving great news about Audrey's condition, and the happiness and gratitude would overflow. At the same time, another family might be hammered with tragic news about their child, and a sense of guilt would weigh me down. I really fought with these two emotions simultaneously. How could I feel guilty that Audrey would be doing well, after everything she had already been through? So I would try somehow to hang on to my appreciation for our circumstances, as I empathized with and tried to comfort other families with heartbreaking situations. And they would do the same for us on days when the news was reversed. We came to know and love these families, as we practically lived together for extended times, while sharing each other's victories and struggles, crying and laughing together over a pizza! We formed an inevitable bond with them.

I still struggle with these two emotions. I found a journal entry I made about a month after Audrey returned home from her transplant:

"A dear friend passed away, after fighting and struggling since her transplant. My heart has been breaking for her family. We walked through this new experience together with separate and very different destinations. As we are rejoicing, they are grieving, as we are sharing our good news with others, they are bearing their saddening news and feel the pain every time they have to talk about it.

As I walk the halls of the Med Center, I am eerily reminded of the anguish we two families felt so often day in and day out. I see how far we have come, and I almost forget that we, too, came very close to suffering loss. And then a certain spot or room or familiar face reminds me of our friend and conversations shared with her mom; and I am quickly and painfully reminded that it all really transpired - for both families - and her ending has to be the thing that brings me back to our reality.

I am back in this twisted conflict of emotion: Gratitude for our sweet Audrey's life - for the way God brought her through everything against extreme odds ... Then guilt vies for my emotions, threatening to steal my gratitude and joy, causing me to ask such questions as, 'Why do I deserve my child to be spared?' Such an unfair question, because I don't deserve this anymore than any other parent... And then guilt slyly attacks at a weak moment ... when I'm up at 2:00 a.m. changing a leaking ostomy bag, along with all of the bedding.

God uses that guilt to reinforce the gratitude in my heart for the privilege of being Audrey's mom, for the chance to have her there to change her ostomy bag! It humbles me that we were chosen as her parents - that God saw us fit and capable and strong enough to carry out the task entrusted to us. And I hug her and kiss her multiple times throughout the day, and tell her how much I love her..."

Journal Entry   April 5, 2008

JSYK

Hang On and Pray Like the Dickens!

I went through stages when I was too numb to pray, and reading scripture and singing in worship were more than I could bear; I would just get too emotional and weepy. I would then reach a phase where I was capable of praying, and would find comfort in reading about the peace found in seeking after the Lord, and about the way trials and hardships strengthen and mold us into better people; how He uses both difficult times and joyful times to bless us and to use us for His purpose.

If you do read the Bible, write down some of your favorite verses on index cards to put up in "your corner" of the hospital room. Add some cards with favorite quotes that might inspire or encourage you.

Or ask a friend to do this for you. Someone would *love* to do something like this for you! You may find solace in taking time to pray or meditate, to focus on things that *are* going right - things as simple as the cafeteria having your favorite Danish that morning, your child having his favorite nurse today, finding a convenient parking spot!

I understand that this is an extremely rough and emotional journey for you. We've been there. And you may wonder if you will make it through to the other side. You may fear the future and find it insurmountable. One of the best ways I learned to get through our experience was to take it one day at a time, and not to look or think too far ahead. I'd like to share with you a couple of analogies that inspired me in our most difficult times.

A Day at a Time...

Morning Glories –

One of my favorite summer flowers is the morning glory. You plant a seed early in the spring, and enjoy shoots of green fairly soon after. The green continues to grow and leaf out, then begins wrapping itself around a trellis or anything in its path. It grows and grows ... and you wait and wait for a flower to bud out. The plant climbs for all its worth as far as it pleases; and still you wait for any sign of blossoms... and they don't appear.

Finally, halfway through the season, the vine starts to fill with buds, and one morning it is veiled in vibrant flowers! Those flowers last only a day and they are gone. But the next morning, you are greeted with another shower of striking blooms raising their heads to the sun. You can depend on that faithful vine to provide you with a palette of color morning after morning for the rest of the season ... until the first frost.

The Old Testament describes the mercies of God: *"... They (His compassions) are new every morning..." (Taken from Lamentations 3:22,23).* Just like those blooms on the morning glory vine, the Lord gives us just what we need for the day, and the next morning He is there to provide mercy, wisdom, and strength we need for the next twenty-four hours. *"Do not be concerned for tomorrow, each day has enough trouble of its own." (Taken from Matthew 6:34)*

Manna –

The other analogy has helped me to keep daily concerns in perspective. It's the story of the Israelites on their escape journey from Egypt. When they reached the desert, they had no food supply and water was scarce. Each morning, God supplied for them wafers, called manna, which were full of the nutrition they needed for the day. Their instructions were to not save any of the manna for the next day. When they tried, the day-old manna was no good; it had spoiled. God promised to provide their food supply daily, and He delivered without missing a day.

These examples are rich with gems that challenge and encourage - they teach on waiting and hope, perseverance and faith. Perhaps they will provide you a little inspiration for yourself, some strength and wisdom that will get *you* from one day to the next. I find it interesting that in the Spanish language, the term *"esperar"* is used not only for both "wait" and "hope", but also for *"expect!"* Waiting and hoping with expectation ... *That's* something to strive for!

A Step at a Time...

Taking a day at a time also calls for taking a step at a time. You may feel as though you are drowning in your circumstances – worry and fear for your child, receiving disheartening news, exhaustion, stretching yourself amongst all of your responsibilities and the people who depend on you ... whatever it may be for you.

I have often heard that in this situation the best thing to do is the next *right* thing. Make a phone call that has been on your list, give your child her bath, straighten up her hospital room, do a load of laundry, go take a nap. Maybe it means taking a walk in a quiet park or taking time that evening to write in your journal to sort out your thoughts instead of surfing the internet; work on a puzzle or read a good book for a little distraction.

If you are struggling with your circumstances and don't know which way to turn, try writing down three simple things to do the next day. Doing this might help you feel like you are moving forward and have a plan. It can also reinstate to you an element of control in a situation that seems to be spinning *out* of control.

You will feel more capable of facing the ordeal if you take one step, and then another, and then another. Don't look farther ahead than you need to. Deal with one issue at a time, taking care of one necessary task at a time.

An example of taking the next step in unimaginable circumstances for us was when it became evident that Audrey's bowels were not going to heal, which meant a successful organ transplant or probable death. At the time, the survival rate for small bowel transplants was fifty percent. These were not great figures for us to base our hope on – but they were the facts – facts we could not change. We followed some steps that were recommended by PICU staff members and the organ transplant team:

1.   The first step for me was to go home and lie on my bed and wail. I cried like I had never cried before – crying out and pleading to God for a miracle, crying rivers of tears ... After an hour or two, I was able to get up, return to the hospital and take the next step.

2. The next step was to sit down with the PICU staff and make a plan. It offered a venue for my husband and I to focus on something other than our circumstances – a plan to *help* us in our circumstances. This step gave us a perspective of purpose and helped us to not despair. Having a plan was like having a lantern that could lead us out of a deep, dark cavern.

3. Then we carried out the steps in the plan. As recommended, we met with the psychologist in the PICU at Children's Hospital where Audrey was inpatient at the time. We counseled with him on several occasions (*don't underestimate the value of counseling through a difficult situation*).

4. Per the recommendations of the PICU team, we also met with our personal physician to see about prescriptions for an anti-depressant to also help us through the trying process of transplant.

5. We met with a psychologist at the Nebraska Medical Center to be interviewed and then to be administered a test required for all caregivers of organ transplant recipients.

6. We made a trip via ambulance from Children's Hospital to the Med Center for Audrey to be evaluated as a possible candidate for an organ transplant.

7. We prepared for discharge from Children's Hospital, to return home and wait for the next phase - that of organ transplantation at the Med Center.

These steps were far from easy, but very necessary. They, collectively, were a means to an end, and they kept our focus on the plan and not on the problem. Carrying out a plan, step by step, to deal with a challenge can help keep you from being overwhelmed, bogged down, and paralyzed with fear.

Having a Plan and Executing It -

We then readjusted to life and to a new routine in our own home and waited for the call. But during that period of time, we had responsibilities to manage Audrey's care ourselves and to keep her healthy, so she would be ready for her surgery. Her care was intensive, but it kept us preoccupied from thinking about that which lay ahead of us.

We had the duty of managing the wound vac on her abdomen. Her bowels had become like a sieve, and the only way to keep her from becoming septic was to dress her belly with a wound vac, which suctioned all of the toxins and waste from her body cavity. We had to make sure the pump was functioning properly, that the collection canisters were changed out when needed, and that her dressing change was performed on schedule and correctly. It was a constant fight to keep all of this working as it should, and we had to continuously problem-solve and get creative, or the results could have been disastrous for her.

Audrey wasn't eating and so we also had her TPN care to manage - making sure her TPN pump was functioning properly, keeping her central line free from infection, and performing dressing changes at the insertion site. She had to withstand numerous forms of adhesive being pulled off of her skin with every dressing change ... between the wound vac and the central line, these happened at least every couple of days!

Did I mention that my husband was called to work out of town during most of this period of time? One snowy day, Audrey's wound vac dressing needed to be changed. The home health nurses couldn't get there, and I had to do it myself. Generally, it required at least *two* sets of hands, and ideally *three* sets of hands to change her dressing. I prepped all of the supplies and then gave Audrey and myself a pep talk. I told her that I needed her help if we were going to get that dressing changed. So she held supplies for me, she even applied pressure with gauze to the "geysers" shooting out of her belly *(that's what we nicknamed the holes in her bowel!)*, so that I could get the work done as quickly and effectively as possible. After the task was finally completed, my shoulder muscles just ached from so much tension!

All of this was taxing and meticulous work. When I look back, I wonder how in the world we did it. But these hoops and hurdles that we had to jump through *and* over on a daily basis, though stressful beyond words, served in their own ways to get us to the transplant. I didn't have time to think about her transplant or the risks, or all of the things that could go terribly wrong. The Lord spared me from undue worry by giving me a task that was more than I thought I could handle. I had no choice but to go through the motions of taking care of her, and that is all I had the time or energy to focus on. We approached each day and each task one at a time, one step after the other.

Stories of valor, surviving hardships and overcoming odds really move me. I think that is why I appreciate war movies. I can do without the violence, the suffering, or the carnage. What inspires me in these stories is the courage and the commitment, the drive and the spirit of soldiers who have banded together to carry out a mission, no matter what it may cost them personally. I see fear in their eyes, but that fear is overshadowed by something stronger that carries them through. They have a plan of action and tunnel vision as they charge forward, dedicated to a cause that is bigger than themselves.

The hardships and trials of others challenge me to meet my *own* troubles head on and to deal with them. They generally cause me to count my blessings, too! Things could always be worse! I overheard my uncle on a phone call with a friend *(I wasn't eavesdropping, just passing by!)*. This was his response to his friend: *"Catastrophe? There are no catastrophes, only opportunities to grow!"* It stuck with me.

Just for kicks, I'll share with you another entry I made along the way; it's a good representation of my state of mind six months into another long admission!

> *"A surgery resident or student shows up at six in the morning, and I am now empowered with a new boldness to order them out of the room and not disturb my sleeping daughter. This is almost worse - I am now considering how to better arrange the furniture in the waiting room. I already arrange and straighten the books on the shelves. I have them all organized just the way I like them!"*

> *Journal Entry   November 2, 2006*

JSYK

"Just so You Know..."

Value a sense of humor! If you don't already have a sense of humor, I highly recommend that you acquire one! Just like counting your blessings, finding some humor in your day is good for the soul. If you look for it you will find it!

A happiness recipe that works for me is balancing stress and bad news with equal parts prayer and gratitude, inspiration and humor, good coffee and dark chocolate!

Journal about your emotional rollercoaster!

What are some of your emotional struggles right now?

_____

_____

_____

_____

What are some initial steps you can take to help deal with one of these struggles?

_____

_____

_____

_____

_____

_____

_____

_____

How can these steps help with the bigger picture?

_____

_____

_____

_____

_____

_____

_____

_____

_____

_____

_____

_____

_____

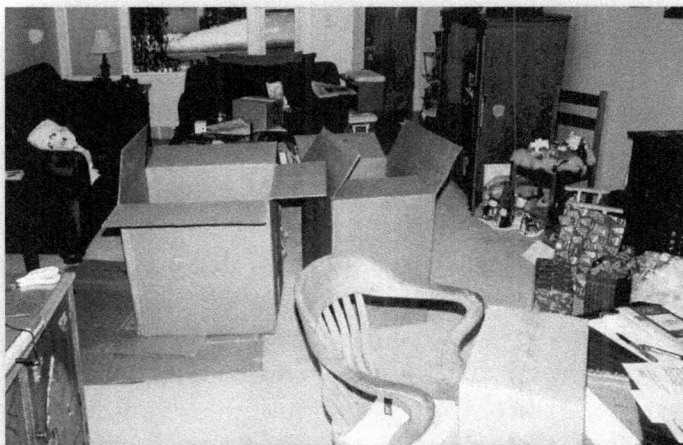

Chapter 12

Adjusting to Life Back at Home

"After living in the hospital for six months, and the subject of going home was addressed, I almost panicked!"

"Oh, You Might Need Some Help?"

I have *heard* of families who bring home newborns, and for the first couple of weeks are surrounded by a force of troops who provide them with hot meals, offer to do laundry and clean house. Grandparents may come to help with the care of the baby and the other children, allowing the new mom time to catch up on sleep and to regain her strength. There are new routines and responsibilities to get used to, and this team of supporters helps the family to adjust to their new life.

If your child requires special care after returning home from the hospital, you *will* have a few adjustments to make. There may be pumps to learn how to operate, a new feeding system to manage, a collection of meds to administer - with a whole schedule of their own, I might add! You may have physical or occupational therapy exercises to carry out with your child. You may have a living room full of supplies that you have to find some place to store! You may be required to rise several times in the night to tend to certain cares. And reality tells me there won't be an army of people waiting to greet you when you walk through the door, ready to go to work to help set up your new routine or relieve you from duty when you need a little shut-eye!

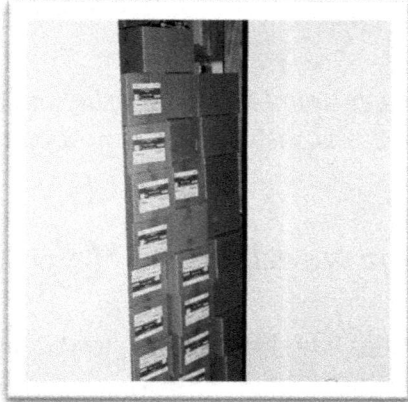

Some boxes took up residency in our kitchen until I figured out where to put them!

Helpers To the Rescue!

One of my missions in life is to establish more integral family support, emotional and physical, for families taking home a loved one who will need ongoing and intensive home health care. In the meantime, I would like to offer some suggestions of how others can help a family in this way. If people offer to help you out, accept their goodwill, knowing that someday you may have the opportunity to do the same thing for another family.

There are myriad ways that family and friends can help you as you return home. If they offer, here are some ideas to make them feel useful and to preserve your sanity:

Meet you at home and help feed/put the kids to bed while you figure out your new pumps, your new med and feeding schedule - allowing you *locate* all of your meds and supplies, *hook up* the pumps, administer the feedings and meds, do a needed dressing change, find space in your fridge for the *mound* of TPN bags, formula, or meds!

A trusted friend with whom your child is familiar could soothe her with books, art projects, games, etc. to help calm her in all the chaos. She may be happy to be back home, but it is still an adjustment to surroundings and routines that were different from what she experienced in the hospital. The adjustment will be greater, also, the longer the period of time that she spent in the hospital. She'll probably even be missing her nurses!

The next day, other friends might bring in a hot meal, totes, organizing drawers, storage containers for formula, cups or scoops with the right measurements or volumes to mix up formula, etc. Then they might help you organize all of your supplies - drawers and storage for dressing supplies and incontinence; medicinal supplies such as syringes, med cups and alcohol wipes; meds and formulas, etc. They could help you find a place for everything and put everything in its place!

Others might help you with meals, cleaning, and catching up on laundry for a week or two - you may find it difficult to keep up with all of this for awhile!

The computer whiz of the group could set up some charts to help you get organized and plan out your schedule of cares and meds! At the end of this chapter, you will find copies of some of my charts that perhaps will be useful to you.

The filing queen may help you organize a system in a portable tote of all of the sheets you brought home from the hospital; home health care information and forms; insurance and medical statements; a file for each department or doctor with related papers pertaining to exams, tests, vaccinations, etc.; other papers and reference sheets from various departments, i.e. physical or occupational therapy, Child Life, etc.

This, my friend, is the first battle to win - getting organized and planning out your schedule. You may have a lot of cares to keep up with, and it will help to have a visual aid to refer to. As a side note, I kept my cares and med schedule sheets on the fridge; and on the dining room table, my folder of her I's & O's sheets (input/output that I had to document). Inside this folder, as I mentioned in a previous chapter, I taped business cards of doctors and specialists, or listed important and frequently accessed numbers, i.e. home health-supplies, pharmacy, etc. Find what works for you!

Tips For Your New Duty as "Supplies Manager"!

May I make one suggestion concerning supplies? If there are important items you access on a regular basis, i.e. dressing supplies, formula or TPN items, meds ... keep a realistic supply in portable totes with secure lids. This is for convenience and safety. If you would ever need to evacuate in an emergency, you can grab your totes that are already packed. Or if you are simply packing for a trip, you can *grab your totes!* And you are less likely to leave something valuable behind!

This is also a convenient way to transport your supplies to another room in the house. At the end of the book, along with charts, is an example of a packing list that I referred to often. If you manage your lists/charts on a computer rather than hand writing them, you will find it much more efficient and convenient, because you will likely be modifying them frequently, as your child's needs or care requirements change.

Maintaining an Accurate Record of Meds –

I have addressed this before, but it bears mentioning again, perhaps a couple more times: Keep a current list of your child's meds with you at all times - in your purse, or your home medical folder that you may carry with you. Make sure to include the "mil equivalents" of each dosage (the proper concentration of the drug). The list of medications you are given at discharge will have this information.

All medical facilities refer to mil equivalents when measuring the proper dose of a medicine. For example, should you need to go to the emergency room, this information will be necessary if your child is admitted and administered his meds from the hospital's pharmacy. If your child has other medications that are administered in a clinic or elsewhere, it would be helpful if you included these in your records.

Anytime you enter a clinic or doctor's office, including dentists and eye doctors, the office will want to document all medications your child is taking and the accurate dosage. I found it helpful to create a med chart on the computer, which made for easy updating.

I also keep a folder of outdated charts for reference, should I ever need them. This means that I have on file any medications that Audrey has ever been administered as an outpatient, along with the dates she was on those medications.

I have also recommended keeping a record of any meds *ever* administered, including meds given while in the hospital: sedatives, pain medications, anesthesia, etc. Remember to note the dates administered, the purpose of the meds and any side effects. This may be helpful information in the future. For example, after witnessing some disturbing side effects that Audrey displayed with certain sedatives, we "nixed" those sedatives from our list of approved medications!

Also noted in her chart was the recommended dosing for other sedatives and pain relievers, as she had built up such a tolerance to the effects of the drug. At one point, after she was given a medication to make her drowsy for a procedure, *I* was the one to fall asleep while she remained bright-eyed and bushy-tailed!

JSYK

A New Routine, an Exhausting Schedule, Different Surroundings, a Huge Responsibility...

I almost panicked at the thought of going home, because after six long months, the *hospital* had become home! We had our routine, our place, and support for Audrey's needed medical care. I would now be solely responsible for her medical care. We would have to establish a new routine. It meant "moving" and "unpacking" *again*!

Post-Traumatic Stress Syndrome –
(Or Being Just Plain Tired!)

As a disclaimer, this condition was self-diagnosed. Perhaps I am being overly dramatic about the "traumatic." I only know that the couple of years post-transplant, I was still a little traumatized from circumstances that I had been faced with in the heat of battle. It seems that when we were in the thick of it, it was about pure survival. Fear and emotion were put on the back burner; I kept them inside, and really didn't know how to deal with a lot of my emotion! I think my body and mind just needed time to recover, to get readjusted to what is supposed to be a "normal" life at home, to regain my strength after years of little sleep and lots of anxiety!

As I previously mentioned, had I known what was ahead of us, I would have sought counseling from the beginning, and followed through with it to the end. But who could have predicted our lot? Our ordeal dragged on for about five years! We had additional issues and challenges, as well, in our lives that contributed to the anxiety. Just having someone who acts as a sounding board can prompt you to release thoughts and feelings you might otherwise internalize, providing you with advice and encouragement from an "outside source!" If you keep negative energy inside, it magnifies the stress and eats away at your overall well-being.

It has now been a fair amount of time since Audrey has needed any home medical care, to speak of, and I feel like I am just now *almost* recuperated from the toll those five years took - physically, emotionally, psychologically, spiritually. I still get up at night to take her to the restroom, but her general care is that of a normal child. She has daily maintenance drugs to take, and we have to monitor her blood pressure, plus monthly or bimonthly lab work. And because she has a suppressed immune system, I try to keep her as germ free as I can without placing her in isolation! This responsibility weighs heavily on me.

For the longest time, I struggled with fatigue and minor symptoms of depression. I felt lazy when I was so tired and ... well, overwhelmed! I had a difficult time getting it together due to a combination of stress, tiredness, and so much to keep up with. It is just plain hard, *to say the least*, to get it together when you are already tired and overtaxed! It's a challenge to concentrate and think of what to do next, and sometimes difficult to build up your momentum. You might get frustrated that you can't seem to reach your previous energy level and gumption it takes to *get* organized and accomplish what needs to be done!

You may come home from the hospital already exhausted, and with this daunting responsibility awaiting you. The tiredness may continue for awhile until you settle into a routine and get your life and responsibilities in order. My advice is to rest when you can. Try to reach a balance of work and rest. If you seem to require more sleep than you used to, don't fight it. Your body will recover or compensate . . . *someday!* If you do have to get up during the night to empty an ostomy bag or administer feedings or meds, check on tubing, monitors, etc., then you probably aren't getting restful sleep.

Call in the forces when you need to!
Grandma, Aunt, Friend, Neighbor...Home Health Care

During one stint at home, I called the "powers that be" in desperation, asking for some nursing help. Audrey's condition was requiring almost hourly 'round-the-clock care. Dallas was working out of town, and so I was on my own. I laid out for them her care plan and schedule, and they were very understanding, sending in reinforcements within a reasonable time. This is help that I should have been offered prior to discharge, but the level of care Audrey would need going home wasn't recognized by the hospital staff.

If only the nurse is consulted regarding the amount of care, the staff will overlook all of the many hats you will wear at home besides just "home nurse". It is important to recognize that once the patient is home, caregiving is a whole new ball game!

You will become the secretary to schedule all of the follow-up appointments: doctors' visits, lab visits, perhaps physical and occupational therapy schedules. You will also take on the role of pharmacy technician - maintaining the inventory of all the medications, ordering as needed, drawing them up, and keeping syringes washed and stocked. The nurses generally receive medications already drawn up, and don't have to worry about keeping them stocked.

You will also become the "Inventory Control Clerk", as you maintain your inventory of assorted supplies, order as needed, and then organize supplies as you receive them. At home, powdered formula will not arrive already measured and premixed. On the hospital floor, the formula containers are tossed when empty - there are no dishes to be done.

When a patient is hungry, food service is contacted, who then delivers the meal and later picks up the tray. When the linens are continually soiled from spits, leaking ostomy bags, leaking feeding and drainage tubes, leaking wounds, leaking diapers, etc. *(our lives were about leaks for several years!)*, housekeeping whisks it away to be washed in another department, *sometimes off site!*

At home, I covered both day and night shifts - rising in the night to refill enteral feeds, administer an IV antibiotic, change diapers, change linens from the aforementioned "leaks", empty an ostomy bag, *change* the ostomy bag, tend to an alarming TPN pump, med pump, feeding pump, wound vac ...

Also, in the midst of nursing care, I had to remember that I was also a mom and a wife. I needed to muster time and energy to do important "mom" things, and to be a wife to my husband, and to try and keep up the house and yard, grocery shopping and errands, etc.

I don't mean to underestimate all of the responsibilities and duties nurses have to juggle. My point is that, from experience, more consideration could be given to the responsibility of the home health care that will rest on the parents' shoulders.

Making Home Health a Part of Your Team-

Once you know that discharge from the hospital is in the works, start considering what it will involve and mean for you. If continued care is needed at home, find out what home health care organization will oversee the care. Ask questions regarding what this care will require, and make sure insurance is approved. Check also with your insurance provider to see what they may cover in nursing hours. If coverage is denied, and help is needed, pursue it. Don't take "no" for an answer until all of your options are exhausted.

Plan Ahead and Voice Your Needs!

Will service include visits from nurses? Do *you* feel you need nursing assistance, especially at the beginning, as you are getting accustomed to new responsibilities and routines? Have a staff member familiar with home health care sit down with you and make an honest evaluation of the care of your child, so you know whether you might need help or not. The liaison that you have cornered and recruited by now *(per my suggestion in Chapter 5)* should be able to help you with this. Maybe together you can write out a home care plan and schedule. This person could probably help you think of the responsibilities you will have as the sole caregiver at home, and make recommendations regarding nursing assistance.

Assess your situation and consider honestly whether you may need a little help for a short while or long while. You are the only one who will be able to accurately determine in what capacity you may need assistance. It might require a call to your home health provider by *you*, to see about setting up some nursing care, if this wasn't taken care of prior to discharge. These needs should be addressed for you as you prepare for discharge, but in my experience, home health care assistance usually got overlooked. It would then be addressed after we arrived home. The disadvantage to this is that it generally takes a couple of weeks to get home health care in place. Those first couple weeks are when you need the most help!

Will your child be going home on equipment? Will the home equipment be different from that which is used in the hospital? How soon will you be introduced to these pumps or machines? It would be worth asking if you could use them in the hospital for at least twenty-four hours prior to discharge to familiarize yourself with their operation and functions. We were given a med pump the afternoon of discharge, and at 11:30 that night, when it wasn't functioning correctly, we had to call our home health team, who then had to deliver a new one in the middle of the night!

Do you have all the "nonessential" medical supplies that your home health organization may not provide, such as measuring and mixing containers for formula? Do you have the proper tools for measuring formula or other liquids with the right quantity and standards of measure, i.e. "mililiters" or "ounces"? If you do have to mix formula or any other supplement at home, you might review instructions with a nurse or home health staff member ahead of time, just in case you have any questions about the mixing, converting or figuring to acquire the correct measurements and dilutions.

Novice vs. Veteran Home Health Care Parent-

The other consideration is the level of experience of the parents or other primary caregivers. If you are new to home health care, you should be lent more support until you feel comfortable with the tasks and routine required of you for your child. The day we went home on TPN and a feeding tube, along with a med pump for administering IV antibiotics to Audrey, the home health nurse training me on the med pump commented that they didn't generally send parents home with that much responsibility without nursing assistance. However, being the seasoned home health caregivers that we were, what was one more pump?!

As she shared this with me, I recalled with a smile the day we took Audrey home from the NICU for the first time. She was over nine months old, my first child, and *I*, for the first time, was responsible for her care, *including* medical care. She went home with a central line that we had to dress, and TPN nutrition that I had to manage. I honestly didn't know if I was up to the task! I was scared out of my mind! They trained us on the home equipment the day of discharge, and I stuck my finger with a syringe. I lost it, breaking into tears and thinking, *"I can't do this! This is beyond me!"* But I rose to the challenge, and found that I *could* do it ... and much more!

JSYK

My Honorary Nursing Degree...

As a young girl, with my entire future laid out before me, I had dreams of what I wanted to do with my life. My best friend, Michele, and I planned to be detectives, and team up with Starsky and Hutch *(or so we thought!)*. A pilot, musician, businesswoman, and social worker were all on the list at some point, too. Funny, but the medical field never even entered my mind! I was squeamish at the sight of blood and smell of vomit and other bodily secretions; injury and trauma just gave me high blood pressure and sent me into a panic! Now after countless secretions, surgeries, injuries, traumas, and other clinical challenges, I am receiving regular email advertisements for nursing schools! Is that some kind of a cruel joke?

So, since I got roped into this training totally against my will, and mastered the skills set in my lap, I hereby willfully grant myself an honorary nursing degree! I don't plan to enroll in nursing school; it's a noble step, but not for me. I don't regret, however, *anything* that I had to do for Audrey! For her it was all worth it. And for myself I found out what I was made of and capable of facing and overcoming. I share my victories for one reason only - to instill confidence in *you* that *you* can do it, too! The Lord gifts us with the strength and courage to confront and conquer!

JSYK

"Just so you know..."

If you are approaching the date for your discharge, you might find it helpful to start making notes of questions and details that you need to address, and with whom you need to address them. Keep a good record of your answers and who your sources were, along with contact information. An issue may arise in which you need to get back in touch with them, or you think of other questions you need to ask them.

Questions:

_____

_____

_____

_____

_____

_____

_____

_____

_____

_____

_____

_____

Contact information to gather:

_____
_____
_____
_____
_____

_____
_____
_____
_____

Supplies to ask home health about or to look for before discharge:

_____ _____
_____ _____
_____ _____
_____ _____
_____ _____
_____ _____
_____ _____
_____ _____

Other issues to discuss directly with home health:

_____

_____

_____

_____

_____

_____

Create a tentative care plan for home, including schedule of meds and cares, and related tasks, i.e. measuring formula, prepping syringes, appointments to schedule, etc.

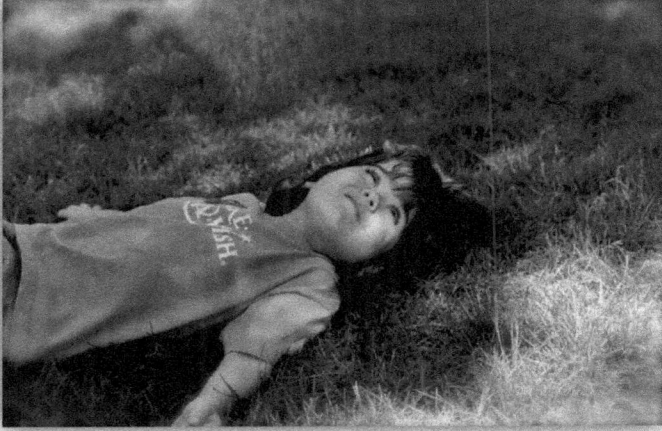

In Summary...

The second year into our story, I had the notion to write a book about our experience, how we made it through, things that helped us... But I didn't know whether I had earned the right to produce such a work - there were other families who had suffered much greater hardship than us, even death; did I really have material worthwhile sharing that would be of any consequence to someone? As I review the contents of *this* book, I wonder whether I have shared too much of our story. Because it really isn't about us or about the events that took place in our lives - events that almost seem unbelievable to us even now. There will always be someone with a grander story, maybe even conveyed in a more spellbinding manner. I simply share a part of ours so that you know someone else who has been through the fire, survived, and is here to encourage you through it.

My challenge to you is to face your situation and be strong when you can; become a problem solver for the sake of your loved one and for others in the same situation; find a shoulder to lean on when you need to; glean advice from whatever sources you can.

I'd like to close with an update that I sent via email a few years ago to our supporters, to those who rallied with us during Audrey's struggles. It really is more of a reflection than news of Audrey's progress. But it sums up how I have been refined, molded, supported, taught, guided, and loved by my Lord, who loves Audrey more than I could ever hope to. Ironically, this was sent just months before we even knew that Audrey would be receiving a transplant:

"This past year, God has been grilling me to be thankful, to be joyful, and to be patient. While such simple truths, they so easily get lost in the grind of daily living or in the middle of a crisis. I've learned a lot about hope in the past few years, so that's a given right now. The sovereignty of our all-powerful God assures me of hope. It's the only predictable and continuous "insurance" we have for Audrey right now.

In times of need and crisis, of discouragement and anxiety, maintaining an attitude of thanksgiving helps to keep you out of the pits. God has nailed me on this one. Every time I start feeling sorry for our situation, He faithfully and promptly puts in my path someone with circumstances far worse than our own. I try daily to put in my mind specific things for which I'm thankful - ways that God has provided for us, blessings that are a part of our everyday lives, the people that God has prompted to reach out to us ... If I put a little effort into it, the list is never ending.

I have never forgotten what I heard a teaching colleague share several years ago, 'Never let anyone rob you of your joy.' The value of joy is that it is self-inflicted. You either allow yourself to be joyful or you don't. Joy is a thermostat for your countenance. It sets the ambience for your attitude, your outlook, your dealings with others, the way you think and act - and react, and live day in and day out. Joy is not a thermometer, it is not intended to read our circumstances and behave accordingly. Joy doesn't decide to take a hiatus on a bad day. It is we who decide such a thing. Joy is a fruit of the Spirit (Gal. 5:22); so as Christians, we are expected to bear the fruit of joy in our lives. We have no excuse!

But God has had to remind me of this, and He is trying to instill this in my soul, until it becomes a part of who I am. It doesn't come naturally just yet, but I am a work in progress! Our daughter has one up on me in this arena. She never lets anything get her down for long. If she sees me having a hard time, she'll ask me, 'Are you happy?' She'll keep asking me until she's satisfied with my answer that, yes, I really am happy. So many people have commented to me about Audrey's joy, and what an inspiration it is to them... 'the joy of the Lord is my strength'(taken from Nehemiah 8:10). This is my daughter's testimony; I want to claim it for my own.

I know that you know that patience doesn't come easily, that it is a virtue! Nothing worth having comes without a price. Patience costs a lot of work, a lot of emotional effort, a lot of biting of the tongue, a lot of waiting, and again a lot of hope. (As I mentioned earlier in this book, "esperar" in Spanish is the verb infinitive for wait, hope, and expect). "Esperanza" means hope, encouragement. Jeremiah 29:11 - 'I know the plans that I have for you', declares the Lord, 'plans for welfare and not for calamity, to give you a future and a hope.' This promise was addressed to a specific group of people, but it is given to us to learn from. Scripture is clear about having trials in our lives, but is just as clear about hope. It also explains how our trials are used to refine us into God's image, how they prepare us for the work in which God will use us, and how they empower us *to help others going through trials. Scripture is also living and active, and this is evidenced in our lives. God is already working out His plan in our family in these very ways.*

When you have a moment, read Malachi 3:1-3. Did you know that a silversmith knows he has held a piece of valuable silver in the refining fire for the right amount of time when he is able to see his reflection in the piece? Hmmm ..."   *(sent May 3, 2007)*

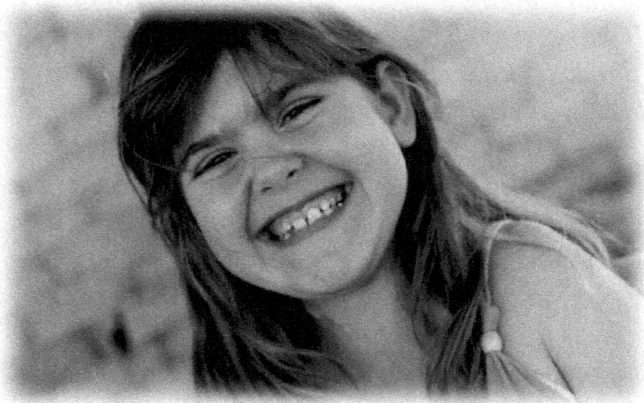

Audrey enjoys life and embraces it and
her loved ones with gusto!

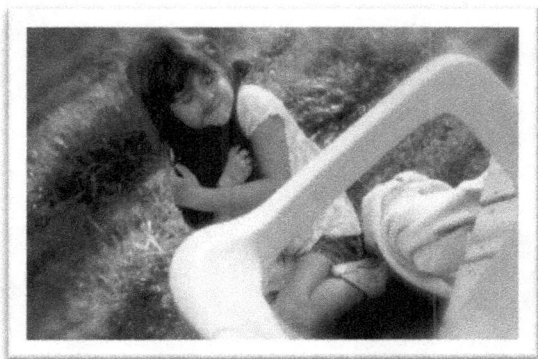

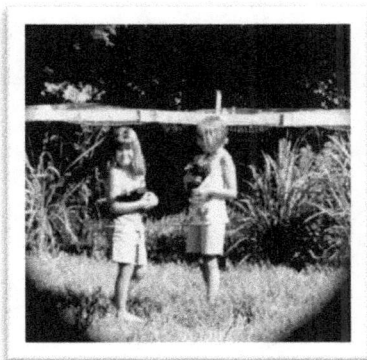

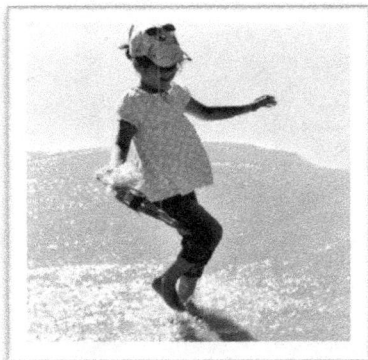

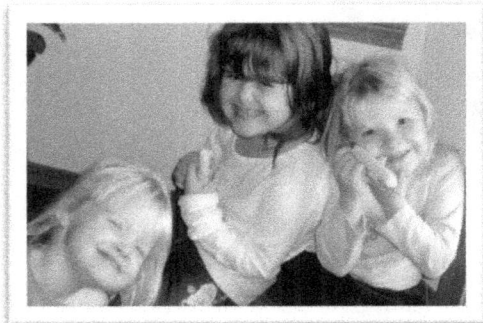

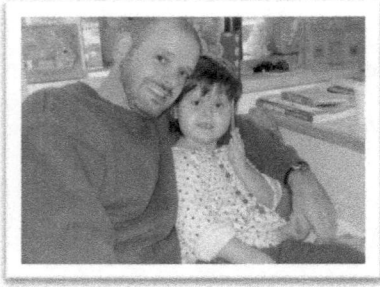

With Dad ...

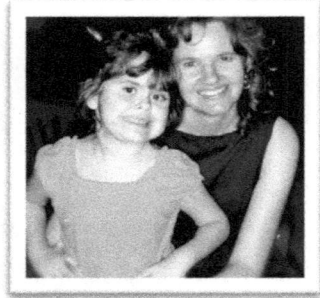

nd Mom

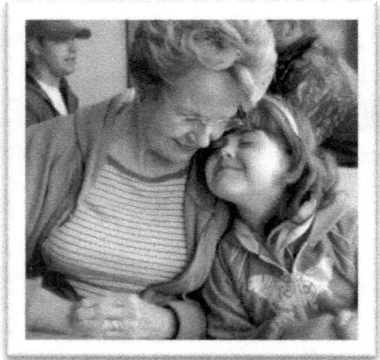

Grandma ...

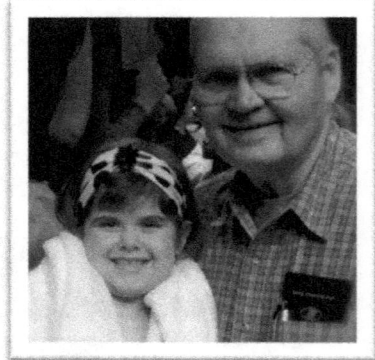

and Grandpa

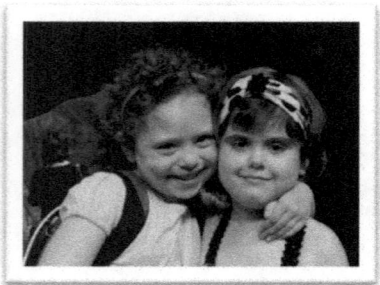

Daisy and Audrey,
"Transplant Twins"

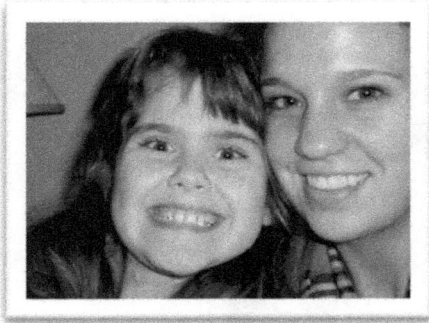

Audrey and her Aunt Tori

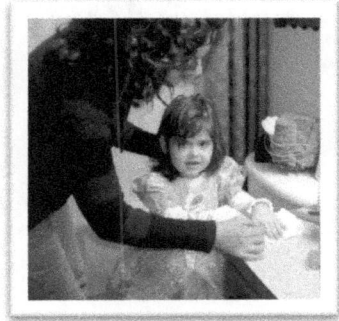

Dolling up for a princess party

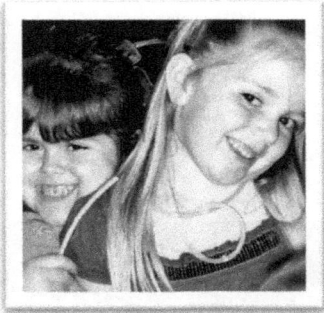

With pal, Lindsey

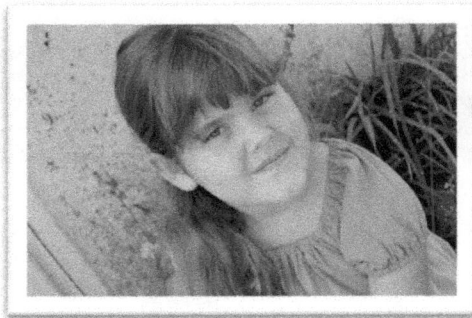

Summer 2012, Age 9

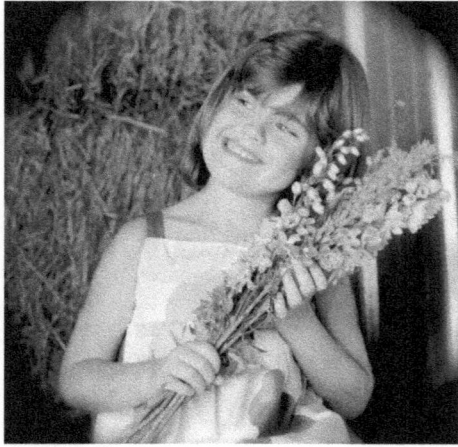

A Country Girl at Heart ...

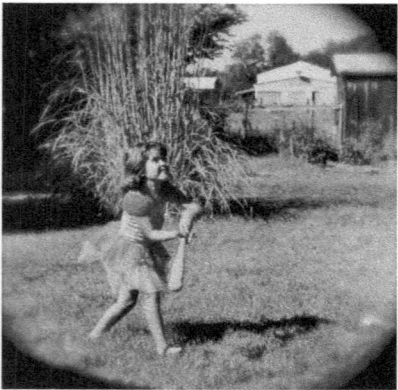

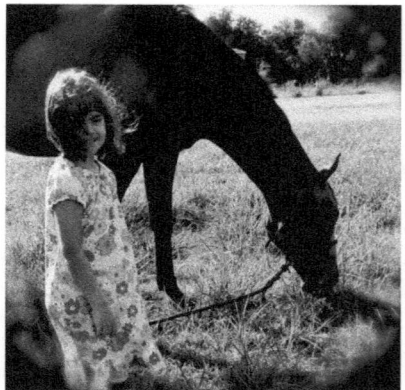

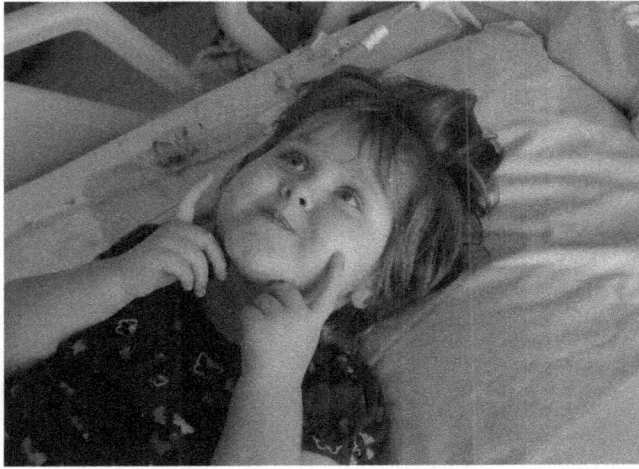

Some Afterthoughts ...

Capturing the Moments on Film -

*O*ne of the last things you will probably think to do or feel like doing is taking your camera out and snapping photos, especially if your child is not doing well. But I encourage you to take pictures. You will want to remember certain things later on; your child, especially if fairly young, will not remember much of his time in the hospital, and may ask a load of questions later on. You will want to share the story, and having photos will help.

   I lived in Colombia, South America, for two years in my mid-twenties. A close friend of mine came to visit me for a few weeks. She advised me to take pictures of the most basic things at first; things that I would soon grow used to, not considering them as novel or unusual or even that interesting as they became a part of my everyday life: The laundry room which was the size of a small half bath, containing only a washing machine and large wash basin, a fold-out ironing board about three feet long, and a clothes line about four feet in length; the public bathrooms whose toilets never had toilet seats and where you had to purchase your own "square" of toilet paper; the buses with the red velvet balled fringe adorning the dashboard; the candle I graded papers by during the nightly blackouts that lasted for about six months.

Take photos of your child's room, her nurses, her machines and pumps, procedures, different areas of the hospital you visit, the view out her window, the playroom, the pharmacy drop that keeps you awake at night! I was always going to video the method of changing her TPN at home ... I got into the routine and it became normal, and I never thought to film when I was in the groove!

I felt strange taking photos of Audrey when she was really sick, photographing her horrible red rash and her ostomy in order to track the progress of healing. I'm so glad I did, though. To me, they are a record of how far she has come. I look at those pictures, and then look at her now ... and remember to be thankful. I also wanted as many pictures as possible during the different stages of her young life in case those were the only tangible memories I would hold later if she didn't pull through.

When we were in flight, on our way to Disney World for Audrey's Make-A-Wish trip, I was reviewing photos in my camera, deleting and prepping the camera for new photos of our exciting adventure. It had been just ten months since Audrey's transplant, and she had only been home a total of about six months. As I reviewed the photos, which were primarily from her hospitalization post-transplant, shots of her most critical moments appeared on the screen: Her bout with Graft vs. Host Disease when her outcome was uncertain; pictures of her sedated and intubated, covered with that nasty red rash and open sores, puffy; her room crowded with IV poles and med pumps, supplies, kidney dialysis equipment...

All of a sudden, it struck me what she had *really* overcome. Sitting beside me on the plane, her face one big smile, I was once again filled with gratitude; and then I'm sure my eyes filled with tears!

JSYK

Audrey enjoys browsing through photos and videos of another time. Most of her first five years of life are documented in this footage! Instead of a baby book, we have pictures and mementos from the hospital. It makes those photos with a spoon in her mouth instead of an NG tube in her nose that much more precious!

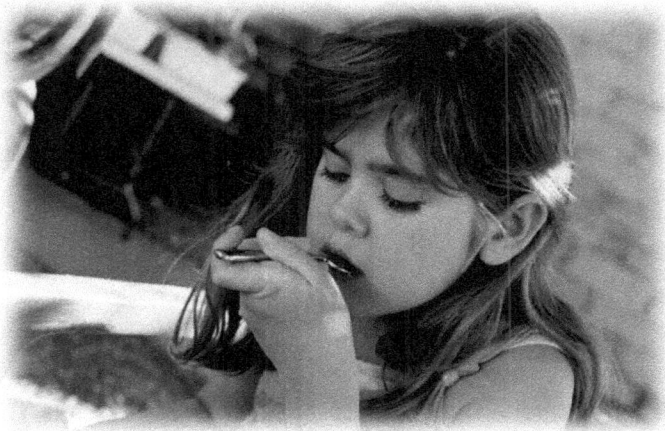

She Kissed Her NG tube "Good-Bye!"

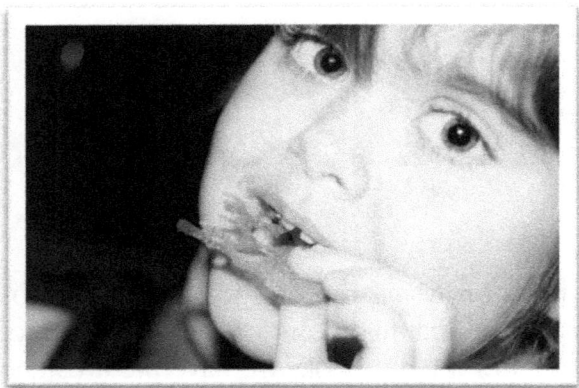

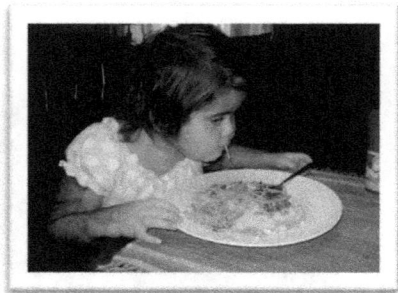

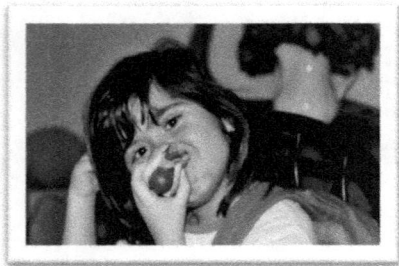

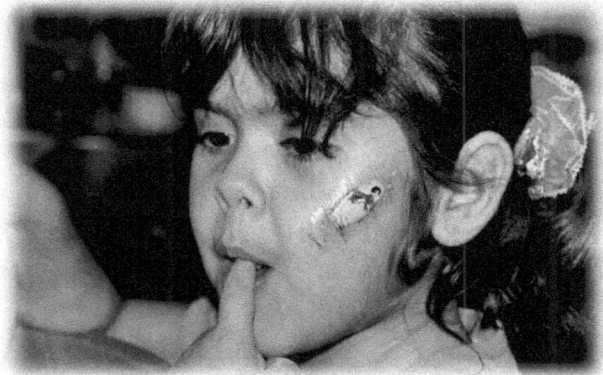

A Picture is Worth a Thousand Words ...

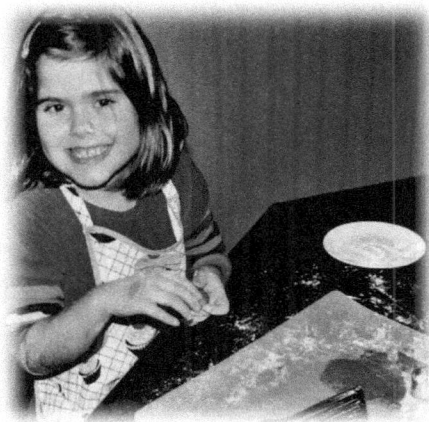

The Importance of Therapy and Exercise-

While we are on the subject of therapy, I'd like to mention the importance of keeping your child's muscles, lungs, and other parts of their body toned and strengthened. It takes very little time for a small body to lose its strength and for its muscles to atrophy.

Your medical team is probably on top of this, and bringing on board those specialists who can help with this. If not, take the initiative yourself to address this issue with your team.

"Just so you know..."

OT stands for Occupational Therapy, and PT stands for Physical Therapy. Occupational Therapy addresses finer motor skills, such as hand strength and coordination, while Physical Therapy is for general strength and endurance, such as muscle toning and use of limbs, expanding lung function, etc.

There are simple exercises that you can even do with your child:

To give his lungs a workout, let him blow bubbles or a whirly gig, or anything else he may enjoy blowing on, such as a little play recorder or kazoo.

Simple play like dressing dolls or throwing a nerf ball into a little basket *(or bedside basin!)* will strengthen weak arms, hands and digits. Tea parties and building with legos or other blocks can be fun and strength building, too. Play also puts some control in the hands of the kiddos, as they choose what to play and how to play it.

They get to pick out the clothes they want to dress their doll in, what they want to create with their blocks, who they would like to invite to their tea party – let them invite their nurse or offer some "tea" to their doctor during rounds – another act in building trust.

Cutting shapes out of paper or tracing shapes on an easel, coloring and drawing, play dough, and playing board games can remedy boredom, while offering some occupational therapy for strengthening.

The "Smiles" Game-

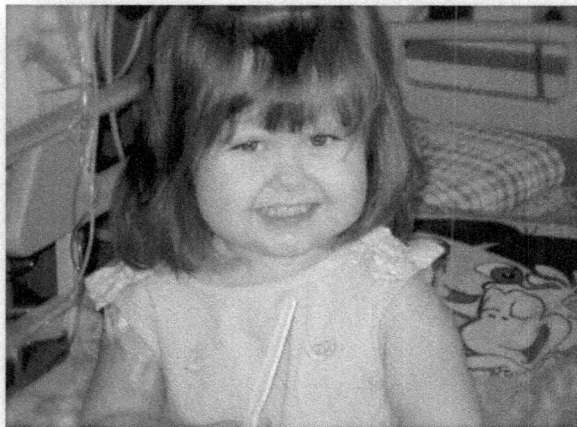

On a good day, we saw lots of smiles!

Try and make the days productive for the sake of everyone's mental health! Think of activities that would be a good distraction from the negative invasions of the day, perhaps a fun game would allow your child to assert herself and be in control of something; some interaction that might provide some needed physical, occupational, or even emotional therapy!

During a stint in the PICU, Audrey was struggling not only physically, but emotionally ... she was mad! She could not get a moment's peace; there was constant activity in her room; every few minutes, a staff member was entering her room to poke, prod, get information, check a pump, etc. You could just see her tense up every time she heard the door open. There was commotion outside her door one day, and she looked at her grandma and asked: "Are they coming for me, Grandma?"

So I created a "smiles" game for her to play. I drew several different silly smiles, one each on a little piece of paper. I attached a paper clip to each smile. I then took a pipe cleaner, bent it into an "L" shape, wrapped an end around a little toy magnet she had, and showed her how she could "fish for smiles". We scattered the smiles all over her bed tray, then with her makeshift fishing pole she tried to catch smiles by grabbing the paperclips with the magnet.

It was not the magic pill to make everything in her world all right again, but it brought a little lift in her spirit. This simple little game also provided some much-needed therapy to her weakened arms and hands.

A Word to the Wise –

If your child isn't in a pediatric hospital, chances are he won't have therapists who are specially trained in working with children. As a result, his therapy sessions may slightly resemble "boot camp!"

If his workouts seem a little harsh or impersonal, take the liberty to suggest activities that are more kid friendly and involve playing. If he's playing, it won't seem like therapy. Throwing a ball or dressing a doll doesn't exactly seem like work to a child! The therapist may even be able to push her patient a little more if he is having fun! What child ever admits that he's tired or sore if he's caught up in fun?

"Splish Splash!"

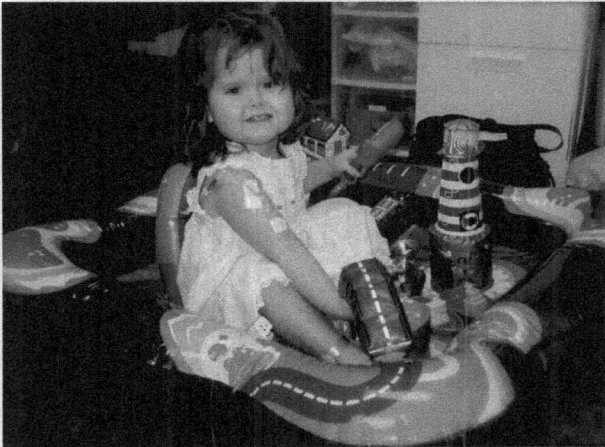

Our friend, Kathy, found this fun shallow pool that Audrey could splash around in without getting her lines wet.

If your child has tubes or lines that prevent him from being able to take a bath, he may still enjoy a little water playtime! Fill a basin of water, bubbles, and toys for him to play with while you give him a sponge bath. Perhaps he'd like to sit on a pillow and stick his feet in to splash around!

If you are giving him sponge baths, see if you can get a couple of warm blankets to wrap him in, so he doesn't get so cold; cover the parts that aren't being washed with a blanket or towel, then as you finish washing a leg or an arm, wrap a warm blanket around them, while you continue with the bath. If you have ever taken a sponge bath, you know how unpleasant they can be and how cold they can make you feel!

Oral Therapy –

If a child has been NPO for a substantial period of time or has had tubes placed down her throat, she may develop an oral aversion. This can cause a child to not want to eat when she is able to. Lack of positive stimulation in the mouth or throat can cause a child to want to avoid a piece of food or even a spoon from being put into her mouth. Different textures of food can seem unpleasant or strange to a child who isn't used to eating. And if she has had to swallow an NG tube or have a vent tube put down her throat, she may be afraid to swallow; if this has been recent, her throat may be sore or tender.

Understanding and awareness will help *you* to help *your child* if she's experiencing this challenge. Our developmental specialist and therapists offered ways to avoid this aversion. They worked with the doctors and surgical team to encourage oral stimulation whenever possible. This included "non-nutritive feedings". This meant that they allowed me to breastfeed Audrey a few times, as long as the milk was being emptied from her stomach before passing into the bowel. She already had an NG tube in place to suction out gastric juices from her stomach, so the surgeons gave me permission to do this. She was allowed to suck on a pacifier, and we would occasionally dip it in sucrose, which can act as a mild pain reliever for infants. As she got older, she was given spongy swabs that she could suck on that had been dipped in water or a mint cream, which acts as a mouth moisturizer.

Involving your children in meal preparation might also be a way to promote their interest in food. There are steps that fit almost any age group, from pouring and stirring to measuring and grating. Kids are more apt to eat something they've had a hand in making. Creating fun meals that *look* enticing is a nonthreatening way to encourage a child to try a bite! Watch some food shows together. There are cooking programs to be enjoyed for every age, interest, and taste – *almost* any hour of the day!

Ask your medical team what you can do to remedy or avoid oral aversion in your child. If you are inspired with ideas of your own, run them by your team. Again, staying proactive will help your child in the short run and the long run!

Bonding Therapy –

Nurses and specialists trained this new mom in bonding with my baby. Our bonding had unique challenges. As mentioned above, Audrey wasn't able to eat for most of her first nine months of life. One of the special ways a mother bonds with her child is by breastfeeding. Besides oral stimulation, non-nutritive feeding allowed us this bonding time.

We were also allowed skin to skin contact, which studies have shown improves the condition of a sick baby. When I couldn't offer Audrey non-nutritive feeding, I could lay her on my chest and offer her emotional support.

Kathy, the developmental specialist, taught me how to give Audrey newborn massages. This was another form of positive touch, to lend nurturing and love and to counteract the negative contact she received from needles *and* X-ray machines *and* tubes *and* wires *and* dressing changes *and...*

Promoting Communication-

As I mentioned before, Audrey suffered from a seizure several weeks after her transplant, leaving her unable to see for a few days and unable to talk for many days. The preschool teacher at the Med Center created some picture pages for her to use so that she could express to us what she wanted, needed, and how she felt. There were pictures of activities and toys, food and drink, images displaying hot or cold, emotions and pain. This wonderful tool allowed Audrey to overcome the communication barrier when she couldn't use words.

You could use a tool like this if your child is in a similar condition and can't talk, or for a younger child who can't express himself very well yet. You could draw simple pictures or recruit Child Life to help you. They probably have clip art or other computer programs to create these pages for you. To make it easier for you, I will list the specific words we displayed with our pictures; the word was displayed above the picture. There were four to six images per page on Audrey's sheets; if there are too many options for a child to consider on each page, it can be overwhelming or frustrating.

Here they are:

Sad	Pain	Mad	Happy

Uncomfortable	Hot	Cold	Sleep/Tired

Play	TV	Color/Book	Drink	Snack

Chair	Bed	Go for a ride

(Picture of wheelchair or wagon)

A blank square was also available for her to draw her own picture – something she might want to add to the list of options!

Tips on Dressing Changes-

As I mentioned in an earlier chapter, we learned a helpful step to removing Audrey's central line dressing. The dressing was a thin, transparent and pliable sheet. One of Audrey's nurses did some experimenting with its removal on her own skin, so she would understand what it feels like. She found that stretching the dressing *outward* as she pulled instead of *upward* was a less aggressive way to remove it; this method was less harsh on the skin and hair.

We also learned that applying warm wet washcloths to a bandage or other dressing site for several minutes is another effective way to loosen the adhesive. Rubbing baby lotion or an oily cream works well on certain dressings. Just be careful to completely remove a cream from the skin if you are applying a new dressing. I would avoid this kind of cream around central line and PICC line sites.

Steps That Worked For Us in Applying an Ostomy–

For any procedure or dressing change, it is a good idea to always have your supplies ready to go, packages open, all within reach before you start. This minimizes anxiety for your child, frees up your hands, and makes for an efficient time saver, so you can *"git 'r done"* as quickly as possible!

For an ostomy change, this should include having your dressing cut to size and connected to bag, ready to apply. Note: We had better success in not cutting our dressing too much bigger than the stoma itself. You don't want it so snug that it rubs the stoma, causing irritation. But if you leave too much space between the stoma and dressing, drainage will seep under the dressing, irritating the skin and loosening the dressing.

To remove bag and prep the skin:

1. Place a warm, slightly soapy washcloth over the adhesive; or let it soak while your child takes a bath.

2. Start lifting gently at a loose corner, applying a soft pressure to the skin with the warm wet cloth as you are lifting the dressing. As needed, gently rub against the exposed adhesive to help lift it.

3. Have gauze ready to help catch drainage from the ostomy as the bag loosens around it.

4. Gently clean skin, making sure that all product and adhesive residue have been removed, and that the skin is clean and completely smooth and dry before applying a new dressing.

5. Lightly sprinkle stomahesive powder on the skin around the stoma that will have the adhesive on it. Fluff out a gauze pad and lightly spread the powder so that the skin is thinly coated, and the powder covers the entire area, with no skin exposed.
   (I liken it to flouring a cake pan! A thin but thorough coat.)

6. Apply no-sting barrier - the swabs provide more controlled application, but the spray is generally less expensive. Make sure that all of the powder application is covered by the no-sting barrier. Allow to dry completely before applying the new dressing.

7. Apply stomahesive paste around stoma if that works well for you. We opted not to use the paste, because it seemed to irritate Audrey's skin, and it was difficult to remove completely when changing the bag - it would irritate her skin that much more when we tried to remove the residue.

8. Apply new bag and dressing, holding your hand over the dressing area for a few minutes. The warmth of your hand will help set the adhesive on the apparatus.

As you find things that work for you, make a note of them to refer to later - either for your benefit or for the benefit of someone else!

Wading through Bills and Statements –

Hospital Costs 101: I had my first crash course in the NICU. For the first month ... *or* two, yellow stickers were accumulating on sheets of paper on Audrey's wall in her little hospital cubicle. I slowly began to notice that if I requested an item, such as a package of gauze, Audrey's nurses and care partners happily obliged me, as they entered a secret password on the keypad of her bedside "toolbox." They would extract the requested item, peel off the yellow sticker, place the sticker on the sheet of paper on the wall, and then hand me the item with a smile! The day the light bulb went on above my head was the day I realized how much this hospital service was costing us!

I then became more cautious about what I requested, weighing carefully the need for an item, or whether I could do without it – a tissue might work just as well as a piece of gauze! I became well acquainted with the supplies identified by yellow stickers, and those other items that *didn't* carry the ever-so-sublime price tag!

The best advice I can give you is to seek out some help to make sense of the cost of your child's hospitalization and related services showing up on your statements. Decoding medical bills can be tricky. They are so complex, making it difficult to read, much less understand all the itemized costs listed or what insurance has paid (if any). A social worker may be able to offer some direction; or go directly to the financial services office. They likely have financial counselors available for patients or patient families.

When multiple bills begin arriving, representing every office that has had a staff member visit or treat your child, get in touch with someone who can help you tackle these one at a time – before you pull your hair out or before you drown in medical debt! Take it from one who has been there! When I communicated with the office sending the bill, we were on much friendlier terms than if I put it off, hoping it would go away. Burying your head in the sand will not solve the dilemma of mounting medical bills!

During one period of too many bills, probably a dozen that needed to be paid yesterday, I made a copy of all our bills and sent them to each of the respective doctors' offices, along with a letter and a plea for understanding. They were all willing to work with me on getting our bills paid off, some of them even reducing the bill when they found out that our insurance no longer covered Audrey because she had reached the lifetime maximum coverage.

If you find yourself in this same position – maxed out coverage, meet with a social worker at the hospital. The social work staff is there, in a way, as a liaison for the patient and his family, to offer help and guidance in these exact circumstances. They are informed of the options available to you, the services to put you in contact with to ensure any aid available for you.

When there is a community of people to help you shoulder your burdens, utilize it! You will not stand up under the weight of the world for long all by yourself! If your child is sick and facing a lengthy hospital stay or intense treatments or home health care, you need your focus and energy available to tend to your child, not to worry about finances - how you will be able to pay for all of the medical care and still keep a roof over your head!

Start with the Following Steps:

1. Gather all of your current medical bills, and delegate a folder
   just for them. Review them one by one; make the necessary
   calls to each office, inform them of your circumstances, and
   ask how they will be willing to work with you. Figure out
   what you can afford monthly toward your total medical costs,
   divide this amount among your bills, and be frank with your
   contacts about what you can afford.

2. Give attention to the older bills first, before they affect your
   credit, but go ahead and make arrangements concerning
   newer bills so they don't affect your credit either. Maybe you
   can't make a payment right away; but as long as you give the
   billing office a time frame of when you might be able to make
   a payment, they likely won't send your bill to collections.

3. Meet with a social worker or financial services at the
   hospital if you need help and guidance sorting through your
   bills and making a payment plan.

4. If you have no insurance coverage, make sure that you are
   informed of your options to help cover your child's medical
   costs. Ask about any state or federal programs that your child
   may qualify for.

Make any notes that might be helpful or questions you need to remember to ask ...

_____

_____

_____

_____

_____

_____

_____

_____

_____

_____

_____

_____

_____

_____

_____

_____

_____

_____

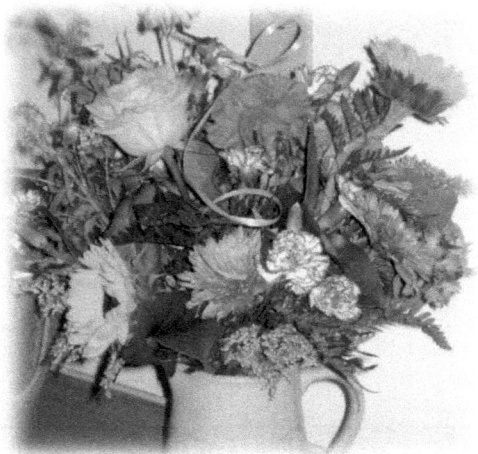

Gift Ideas:

I'd like to share with you some of the greatest gifts Audrey and we received throughout her health challenges and numerous hospitalizations. These might offer you some ideas for your child or other families you happen to meet who could use a bright spot in their day; or if a loved one asks you for some gift ideas, you'll have some thoughts to pass along.

Warm, Soft, Comfortable Linens and P.J.'s. –

There's just something about being hugged by something soft and comfortable when you don't feel good. Audrey received some flannel kitty sheets from her friend, Daisy. They were so soft and cozy, and made her room look so pretty and little girlish! It's all in the details! I suggest dorm-sized sheets to fit the length of the hospital beds.

Fuzzy Socks –

When Audrey couldn't wear normal socks, and the frigid air of the unit made her toes frosty, these over-sized, lusciously soft pink and purple socks were just the ticket. They fit over sat probes, IV's, and therapy boots. They were therapy in and of themselves!

Coloring, Sticker, and Activity Books, "Dot" Markers, Lacing Cards, Puzzles –

Toys and activities that aren't too bulky; you could even include something to store them in – a tote or basket. On one elevator ride, I spotted some women bringing in a wooden crate for a patient. It had been painted in bright colors, with the child's name in bold letters. What a great gift for a child in the hospital – a cheerful, colorful toy box!

Child's Plastic Tray –

You can find these at toy stores. They come with cup holders and storage cubbies. These make a much better bed tray than the hospital ones, which tend to be too high for a child to reach comfortably.

Flowers –

One of the loveliest arrangements I received from friends came in a beautiful ceramic pitcher, holding bright cheery sunflowers front and center, surrounded by wild flowers. Long after the flowers faded, the ceramic piece was a welcoming decorative piece in our room. Now I enjoy it in my kitchen full of dried hydrangeas!

Coffee Shop Gift Card –

This is a wonderful gift for a mom or dad, offering them a "pick-me-up" during a long day...or after a long night!

Gift Baskets –

Filled with items such as a coffee mug, water cup, cocoa, coffees or teas; bath supplies for mom to pamper herself; journal, notepad, and pens.

Magazines for Mom and Dad –

When they are finished, they can donate them to a waiting room.

Utilize the hospital gift shops: They contain treasures!

You may want to keep track of the gifts you have been receiving and who you received them from, such as in your journal - to remember later, plus, as I mentioned before, you can refer to this for thank you cards.

JSYK

Miscellaneous Tip:

Send diapers with your small child on a trip to the OR. Chances are they won't have the size she needs; at least that was my experience!

Useful Medical and Clinical Terms

I thought it a good idea to include a number of basic terms you are likely to hear during your chats with your child's care team. If you are too embarrassed to keep asking them what something means or does, you can first consult your handy vocabulary list that I've provided for you; or you can always look it up online, if you are bound and determined not to ask your nurse for the twentieth time what they're talking about!

General Surgical Terms or Terms Used in the Unit–

Apgar Score: A rating used for evaluating the overall condition of a newborn. This rating considers the following characteristics, and assigns each one a number of zero, one, or two, with a total of ten being a perfect score: Coloring, heart rate, response to touch on the sole of the foot, muscle tone, and breathing.

Central Line: A surgically placed central catheter. Extends into a large vein and is used when IV medications and/or nutrition will be needed for long-term.

Dehiscence/Dehisce *(verb)*: The parting of sutures *(stitches)* at a surgical wound site, resulting from an infection or weakened skin tissue.

Distal: Located away from point of attachment, i.e. *downstream.*

IV (meaning intravenous): IV lines are inserted into a vein, and used to administer medication or fluids for hydrating, including sugars and electrolytes.

NPO: Nothing by mouth, nothing to drink or eat.

OR: Stands for "Operating Room." Medical staff will often refer to surgery as the *"OR."*

PICC Line: A peripherally inserted central catheter. Refers to an IV type of line that is placed into a vein and extends centrally, usually as far as a large vein close to the heart. It is used to deliver medications and/or nutrition into the veins; often used when longer therapy will be needed than a simple IV can last.

TPN/Lipids: TPN stands for total parenteral nutrition, which refers to complete nutrition delivered through an IV or central catheter for nutrition needs, especially when the patient cannot eat. This IV fluid includes sugars, proteins, electrolytes, vitamins and any other needed nutrients. It is also sometimes called **"hyper al"** - hyper alimentation. Lipids are the fats that complete the nutritional package.

Venous: Having to do with veins, i.e. "IV" - intravenous.

Vitals: Health data collected such as heart rate, respiration rate, blood pressure, temperature and pain.

_____

_____

_____

Referring to Heart & Lungs –

Aspirate: To take fluid into the lungs causing difficulty in breathing.

Bradycardia ("Brady"): A low heart rate; may be brief or longer. Can be caused by a variety of medical reasons; frequently seen in premature babies.

Desaturation ("Desat"): A low oxygen level as measured by an oxygen saturation probe. Can be caused by a variety of medical reasons.

Extubate: To remove a tube, especially from the airway after intubation.

Intubate: To place a hollow tube into the airway to allow for machine ventilation/breathing.

Hypertension: Abnormally high blood pressure.

Hypotension: Abnormally low blood pressure.

Room Air: ambient air (air in the room/atmosphere), versus oxygen from an oxygen tank.

(Additional Terms/Notes:)

_____

_____

_____

"Sat" (Oxygen Saturation) Probe/Pulse Oximeter:

A pulse oximeter is commonly placed on a finger or toe to measure the concentration of oxygen in the blood. It is generally referred to as a "sat" probe among medical staff, and is used if the level of oxygen in the blood needs to be monitored, such as when a patient is on a ventilator, is under anesthesia or other sedation, has lung or breathing issues which need to be closely watched. The lungs introduce oxygen from the air we breathe into the blood stream, while extracting or ridding the blood of carbon dioxide. Cells need an ongoing supply of fresh oxygen to survive and to produce energy.

Sedate/Sedation:

To put a patient to sleep by use of medication – dosing with a sedative.

Vent/ventilator:

A mechanical/artificial respirator - a machine that assists patients with breathing or the exchange of carbon dioxide and oxygen.

_____

_____

_____

_____

_____

_____

_____

_____

GI (Gastro Intestinal) Terms -
(referring to digestive system, i.e. stomach & intestines)

Adhesions: Scar tissue; scar tissue "adheres" *(fastens)* to other tissue surrounding it.

Distended: Enlarged or swollen, such as a "distended abdomen."

Drip feeds & Gavages or Boluses: Terms used to describe tube feedings. Drip feeds are slowly and continuously fed into a feeding tube. Gavages or boluses are given over a faster period of time such as 30 to 60 minutes.

Emesis: Vomiting.

Fistula: An abnormal opening at the surface of the skin, generally leading from a wound or hollow organ such as the intestine.

"I's" and "O's" *("Input" and "Output")*: For measuring liquids or food taken in, and measuring that against any output, such as emptying of bladder, bowels, or other form of drainage, such as through an NG tube or other drainage tube.

Motility: Movement, such as movement of the digestive system.

Note ... There are conditions that affect motility, especially for people in the hospital for an extended stay; one is surgery and another is medication. After surgery, medical staff will encourage a patient to get out of bed and start moving as soon as possible, as well as begin decreasing pain medication, as tolerated. The goal is to get the bowels moving again so the patient can begin eating, and also so his lungs don't fill with fluid. This is another danger of a bedbound patient – lack of physical activity can cause a build up of fluid in the lungs, posing a threat for developing pneumonia.

NG/OG/G-tube: Tubes placed in order to suction out the stomach or feed into it. An NG tube is placed from the nose through the esophagus and into the stomach. An OG in inserted into the mouth, through the esophagus and into the stomach. A G-tube or G-button is surgically placed on the abdomen and enters the stomach.

Necrosis: Death of living tissue due to a local injury, i.e. blood loss, corrosion; often occurring in the bowel.

Necrotizing Enterocolitis *(commonly referred to as* **"NEC"***)***:** A bacterial infection and inflammation of the intestines that preemies are especially susceptible to.

Ostomy: An opening created from an area inside the body, primarily from the bowel, for elimination *(emptying)* outside the body into a bag.

Peristalsis: Normal contractions of a muscular organ, such as the bowel or esophagus to move contents down or forward.

Peritoneal Cavity: Also called abdominal cavity, where the organs surrounding the stomach are contained.

Reflux: Backflow, such as reflux in the esophagus, causing the patient to spit up any contents from the stomach.

Upper GI study:
An X-ray study of the esophagus, stomach, and duodenum (first loop of bowel, connecting the stomach to the small intestine). Generally the patient is administered an oral liquid such as barium, a white chalky substance, which can be seen through X-ray to follow the path of the liquid through the digestive system.

Other Terms -

Dialysis: A procedure that takes on the function of the kidneys, such as filtering waste products from the blood. A patient is hooked up to dialysis when his/her kidneys are unable to function properly on their own.

MRI (*"Magnetic Resonance Imaging"*): A procedure involving the use of a large magnetic field *(in place of a conventional X-ray)* for viewing internal parts of the body; more effective in viewing soft tissue, brain and spinal cord, joints and abdomen.

CT Scan: Process of two-dimensional X-rays, revealing soft tissue structures that can't be seen by traditional X-ray. The machine rotates 180 degrees around the patient's body.

Demyelination: Myelin is a white substance made up of proteins and fats that surround and protect nerve cells in the brain; demyelination is the loss or destruction of myelin.

_____

_____

_____

_____

Brigitte D. Crist

These pages offer some charts and other ideas that may prove useful for you. Feel free to adapt and modify any of them for your use!

JSYK

At one point, we left a clipboard outside the door with paper, a pencil, and a large manila envelope with the following note attached. When we wished to be left alone, visitors were able to leave us a message and let us know they had stopped by. *(We still have those notes to read and to remember the wonderful family and friends who stood by us in our darkest hour!)*

Dear Friends,

Thank you for stopping by. We always appreciate visitors! If we have posted a "Do not Disturb" sign, it is because we need to rest or just need some time as a family.

During these times, we hope you understand that we'd be pleased with just a note. You're welcome to leave one on the paper provided. If you prefer a more personal note, feel free to drop it in this envelope.

You are welcome any time to visit Audrey's care page for an update:

(Carepage then listed)

Thank you!

The Crist Family

Below is an example of our inventory of supplies that we needed to keep on hand. This list made for easier ordering. It might serve as a helpful guide for you, as you create your own inventory checklist.

Inventory of Supplies
CHH (Home Health Company)
(Monthly order)

Next order: Aug.10

Enteral Supplies

Formula
Enteral bags

Ostomy Supplies

Bags *(brand name listed)*   1 3/4 in. (ref.# _____) 2 boxes
    (Qty. 10 each)
Wafers (brand name listed) 1 3/4 in. (ref.# _____) 2 boxes
    (Qty. 10 each)
Gauze 4x4 .... 2 boxes
Gloves (medium/nonsterile) ..... 2 boxes
No-sting barrier spray .... 2 bottles

Incontinence

Diapers - Overnights
Pads/Liners - insert in diaper
Chucks *(disposable waterproof pads)*

TPN Supplies

Saline
Alcohol wipes
Betadine wipes

This is a sample packing list that helped me when preparing for any jaunt out of the house, whether it be for 6 hours or several days. (The length of trip dictating the extent of packing, of course!)

Packing List
(Med. Supplies, etc.-for trips)

Enteral Supplies
- ✓ Formula
- ✓ Ice packs
- ✓ Purified water

Meds
- ✓ Syringes
- ✓ Baggies
- ✓ Med cups
- ✓ Pill cutter
- ✓ Vitamins
- ✓ Sodium bicarbonate
- ✓ Med List (frig & non)

Ostomy Supplies
- ✓ Bags & wafers
- ✓ Gauze
- ✓ Gloves
- ✓ No sting barrier spray
- ✓ Syringe for flushing
- ✓ Saline

Incontinence
- ✓ Diapers - Overnights
- ✓ Pads/Liners - insert in diaper
- ✓ "Chucks" *(disposable bed pads)* & diaper wipes

Additional Supplies & Notes:
- ✓ Toiletries
- ✓ Blankets/pads
- ✓ Night light & Monitors
- ✓ Sound machine
- ✓ Disinfectant spray
- ✓ Deodorizer spray
- ✓ Pillow/extra case
- ✓ Trash bags
- ✓ Hand Sanitizer
- ✓ Wipes – for hands & cleaning

This chart can be used for documenting "I's" and "O's"

(Date_____)

Stoma Output	Voids	Food Intake	Fluids

(Cares to note: if output greater than 700 ml in 24 hrs. notify team)

Other Notes ...

_____

_____

_____

_____

_____

_____

The following is a Med Chart that I used; perhaps it will provide some ideas for you as you customize your own chart.

Time	Med	Dose (mg/ml)	Frequency	Purpose	M	T	W	R	F	S	S

Notes:

- I color-coded the font on each row. Visually, it helped me to keep track and spot meds on my list more readily when each row was a different color.
- Remember the mil equivalent *(mg/ml)* is different than the dose – it provides information on the concentration of the medication, much like a liquid drink, i.e. a ratio of lemon juice to water.
- If you have several meds to administer in a day, the last part of this chart may come in handy as you check off each med as you give it. I found this especially helpful if I had meds to give Audrey at varying times throughout the day.
- You may want to put an asterisk beside meds that need to be taken with food, or do your color-coding accordingly.
- Be sure that you understand which of your child's meds shouldn't be taken together, and mark them accordingly. Perhaps these meds should be coded with completely different colors, i.e. shades of red/pink vs. shades of blue/purple.
- If you create a chart like this on the computer, then it will be easy to update. Print out a copy or two for yourself and to hand in at a doctor's office. Or keep a copy in your med folder at home and a copy in your purse so you always have this information with you to provide at a doctor's appointment or in the unfortunate event of a trip to the emergency room.

Make any additional notes of things that come to mind:

_____

_____

_____

_____

_____

_____

_____

_____

_____

_____

_____

_____

_____

_____

_____

_____

_____

_____

Resources to Help Family Members with Coping and Grieving

When God Weeps, by Joni Eareckson Tada and Steven Estes
(A great encouraging read when trying to make sense of difficult circumstances)

If you are grieving the condition of your child or the loss of your child, please don't try to cope with your grief alone. Seek out support from others, whether it be from a pastor or chaplain, or through grief centers that offer support for families, both parents and siblings. You may benefit from meeting with other parents who have lost a child, or who have experienced a similar crisis as yours.

Here are some websites that may be a source of help and encouragement to you:

Centering.org *(resources available for dealing with grief)*

Grievingchildren.org *(support groups available in many communities)*

Compassionatefriends.org *(offering support on many levels)*

Eastonl.com *(an inspirational personal testimony from parents who lost their little boy, Easton; they now support an important cause featured on their website)*
   Note: "l" is the lowercase letter "L", not #1

Abbeyshope.org *(a foundation established by parents who lost their little girl, Abbey; included is their inspirational personal story)*

Carepages.com   Caringbridge.org
(Networking websites intended to share a patient's progress with loved ones)

www.ingramcontent.com/pod-product-compliance
Lightning Source LLC
Chambersburg PA
CBHW031929190326
41519CB00007B/468